A PLUM

HOW WE L

SUZANNE BRAUN LEVINE is a wri... nized authority on women, media matters, and family issues. Editor of *Ms.* magazine from its founding in 1972 until 1989, and editor in chief of the *Columbia Journalism Review*, she currently blogs for *Huff/Post50*, *Next Avenue*, and AARP. This is the third in her series of books about women in Second Adulthood, following *Inventing the Rest of Our Lives* and *Fifty is the New Fifty*. Her other books include *Father Courage* and an oral history of Bella Abzug (with Mary Thom). She also produced a Peabody Award–winning documentary about American women. She has appeared on *Oprah* and the *Today* show, among others, and lectures widely.

Praise for *How We Love Now*

"It's still rare to read anything this thoughtful about our age group, especially about care*giving*. And care*getting*. None of us is too good at that yet."
      —Ellen Goodman, columnist

"[Levine writes about how] going out of the comfort zone and risk-taking are part and parcel of building new intimacies. The road from dependence to independence to interdependence is part of the journey toward finding a peaceful place of reconciliation between 'conflicts of the past and present, work and love, who you are and who you thought you should be.'"
    —Marcia G. Yerman, *The Huffington Post*

"The metaphor I prefer is Suzanne Braun Levine's 'fertile void,' a space of 'unremitting unknowningness.' . . . It is here in the tendrils of the fertile void that something new can begin to sprout—if you surrender to it and don't numb yourself with busyness."
   —Jane Fonda, in *Prime Time: Love, Health, Sex, Fitness, Friendship, Spirit; Making the most of all of your life*

"Suzanne's messages about women in second adulthood are wise, witty, and hopeful. After hearing her, we know that the best is yet to come!"

—Ellyn Cohen, program chair, Rockland, New York, Jewish Family Service

"Her words are confirmation that the physical, emotional, mental, and spiritual changes I am experiencing are not only normal but desirable."

—Audience member, The Transition Network, Columbus, Ohio

"Through research, her own journalistic prowess, and the engaging stories of many women, Levine etches a reassuring picture of the many forms love can take in the lives of women."

—Thelma Reese, ComingofAge.org

"*How We Love Now* is the latest, masterful installment in a trilogy that, I believe, will become the new guidebooks for a second half of life well-lived."

—Marc Freedman, founder of Civic Ventures, author of *The Big Shift*

"*How We Love Now* has the wonderful features of Levine's previous books—the ease with ideas (e.g. brain research), the ability to make them accessible, the parallel ability to see patterns in our lives and still give people their particularity, and the common sense of her advice, its plausibility. My maturing amygdala is lighting up."

—Catharine R. Stimpson, university professor and dean emerita, New York University

"Whether you're single or married, widowed or divorced, this book will remind you of how many opportunities for getting—as well as giving—love already exist in your life, and of the many more that await you."

—Jane Adams, author of *I'm Still Your Mother*

Also by Suzanne Braun Levine

Fifty Is the New Fifty:

Ten Life Lessons for Women in Second Adulthood

Inventing the Rest of Our Lives:

Women in Second Adulthood

Father Courage:

What Happens When Men Put Family First

Bella Abzug:

How One Tough Broad from the Bronx Fought Jim Crow and Joe

McCarthy, Pissed Off Jimmy Carter, Battled for the Rights of Women and

Workers, Rallied Against War and for the Planet, and Shook Up Politics

Along the Way, an oral history *(with Mary Thom)*

HOW WE LOVE NOW

Women Talk About Intimacy After 50

Suzanne Braun Levine

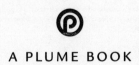

A PLUME BOOK

PLUME
Published by Penguin Group
Penguin Group (USA) Inc., 375 Hudson Street, New York, New York 10014, USA • Penguin Group
(Canada), 90 Eglinton Avenue East, Suite 700, Toronto, Ontario M4P 2Y3, Canada (a division of
Pearson Penguin Canada Inc.) • Penguin Books Ltd, 80 Strand, London WC2R 0RL, England •
Penguin Ireland, 25 St Stephen's Green, Dublin 2, Ireland (a division of Penguin Books Ltd) •
Penguin Group (Australia), 707 Collins Street, Melbourne, Victoria 3008, Australia (a division of
Pearson Australia Group Pty Ltd) • Penguin Books India Pvt Ltd, 11 Community Centre,
Panch1sheel Park, New Delhi – 110 017, India • Penguin Group (NZ), 67 Apollo Drive, Rosedale,
Auckland 0632, New Zealand (a division of Pearson New Zealand Ltd) • Penguin Books,
Rosebank Office Park, 181 Jan Smuts Avenue, Parktown North 2193, South Africa • Penguin China,
B7 Jaiming Center, 27 East Third Ring Road North, Chaoyang
District, Beijing 100020, China

Published by Plume, a member of Penguin Group (USA) Inc. Previously published in a Viking
edition.

First Printing, February 2013
10   9   8   7   6   5   4   3   2   1

Excerpt from "One of the Softer Sorrows of Age" from *Begin Again: Collected Poems* by Grace Paley.
Copyright © 2000 by Grace Paley. Reprinted by permission Farrar, Straus and Giroux, LLC.

 REGISTERED TRADEMARK—MARCA REGISTRADA

The Library of Congress has catalogued the Viking edition as follows:

Levine, Suzanne.
How we love now : sex and the new intimacy in second adulthood / Suzanne Braun Levine.
p. cm.
Includes bibliographical references and index.
ISBN 978-0-670-02322-6 (hc.)
ISBN 978-0-452-29900-9 (pbk.)
1.   Older women.   2.   Older women—Sexual behavior.   3.   Intimacy (Psychology)
4.   Love.   I.   Title.
HQ1059.4.L477 2012
306.7084'6—dc23
2011030172

Printed in the United States of America
Original hardcover design by Alissa Amell

PUBLISHER'S NOTE
While the author has made every effort to provide accurate telephone numbers and Internet addresses
at the time of publication, neither the publisher nor the author assumes any responsibility for errors,
or for changes that occur after publication. Further, the publisher does not have any control over and
does not assume any responsibility for author or third-party Web sites or their content.

For my dear children, Joshua and Joanna

Author's Note

I am immensely grateful to the women who shared their most intimate thoughts and experiences with me. Although many were willing to have their names used in the book, I chose to change all names in order to protect everyone's privacy. In the cases where real names are used, it is because the person is known—or should be known—for their accomplishments or activities.

CONTENTS

Contents

Introduction

Love, Sex, and Unicorns

It has long been my unassailable belief that orgasmic
women can change the world. By this I mean that a
woman who is unfettered sexually is unfettered politically,
socially, economically and she is unstoppable.

—Dell Williams, founder, in 1974, of

Eve's Garden a "Sexuality Boutique" for women,

in her autobiography *Revolution in the Garden*

Since this book was first published I have traveled and talked
to at least as many women (and men) as I did when I was
researching it, and in roughly the same proportion—hundreds
in person, thousands on line.

We talked about the challenges and rewards and surprises
of moving into this totally new stage of life; we compared

notes on the process of reinventing ourselves and how it engenders the kind of energy and creativity and Sturm und Drang we haven't experienced since adolescence. We talked about intimacy and love and taking care of ourselves and others. And we talked about sex.

In my first round of reporting, the big discovery (for me at least) was how many women were having great, uninhibited, inventive sex. And many of those who weren't wanted to. "Despite shriveled orifices and waning hormones, the old girl has never had more juice," I wrote.

Once I put the topic of sex out there by writing about it, I continued to hear countless stories that confirmed that finding, but I was also in for another discovery: the subject itself—that is, older people (including, and especially, ourselves) having sex, wanting sex, seeking advice about sex, or simply being seductively naked—does not come up in otherwise free-wheeling conversations, even among very close friends. Women were amazingly honest and graphic in our phone interviews and even more so online, but not in public and not when they could be identified. Unlike all the other items on the Contents page, this topic was skirted in Q&A's, or workshops, or at book signings. I guessed that those who were doing it were a little sheepish and didn't want to go public. Those who weren't doing it were probably a little cynical and didn't want to hear others sing the praises of a revitalized erotic life. Most were curious but tongue-tied.

In the first chapter of this book, I mention the impulse to "figure out what is going on" that is behind most of my work. That same impulse is behind this effort to amplify the book's original reporting by probing more fully the timidity that surrounds our experience of decidedly untimid sexual experiences.

I found no single explanation for this disconnect in the public/private realm, between what we do or want to do and what we admit to or are willing to talk about. Perhaps it is because we have only gotten halfway to believing that we are entitled to an erotic life after menopause—we go for it, but we don't talk about it. Does talking about it lead to others picturing us doing it, which is embarrassing? Are we still intimidated by unflattering cultural images of older women's bodies and misinformation about older women's sexuality? One woman who was reading my book told me that she removed it from her bedside table and put it in a drawer because she was concerned that the subtitle—*Sex and the New Intimacy in Second Adulthood*, which we have changed in this edition—would shock her housekeeper.

Another explanation may be that for many women, this is the first time in their lives that they can give themselves permission to separate sex and love. Until now we were expected to believe that sex was only approved in combination with love. And reproduction. Women of a certain age no longer have to worry about pregnancy, but nowadays they are also experimenting with disconnecting sex from other requirements as well. Good sex for the fun of it is catching on, but we can't seem to leave the good girl/bad girl baggage at the door.

Whenever I raise this subject in a public forum, someone points out that it is surprising that we have become so shy, since we were the beneficiaries as well as the practitioners of the "sexual revolution." Looking back, though, it is clear to me that all that carrying on wasn't about exploring our own sexuality; it was about experimenting with what we assumed was everyone else's. As in so many other aspects of our lives, each of us now has a second chance to get to the truth about who she is sexually.

When I read about a study that confirmed my findings about sexual activity among older women on *Huff/Post50*, I contributed a comment saying that and, picking up from observation above, added that I was sure "there are a lot of juicy women out there." (I must admit that when I chose the word "juicy," I knew I was being a little provocative.)

"Yes, yes, yes," replied most of the women who joined the discussion, even those who weren't getting any "juicy" sex at the moment. The only negative voices were from a handful of outraged men. They were furious at the suggestion that there were lusty women around, because that most definitely wasn't their experience. "I did encounter one," a man wrote, "and she was riding a Unicorn!" The anxiety behind such bitterness confirms a theme that emerged from my interviews—

when men encounter the least problem in their ability to perform, they give up. They need to listen to what women are saying about the range of erotic possibilities that don't require youthful stamina.

When I began to notice surprising numbers of men—many on their own—in the audiences for my talks, I was afraid I was in for more unicorn comments. Fortunately, I found instead that there was a touching eagerness to have this life experience explained and discussed openly. They knew that if they were looking for truth-telling and support, they would find it among women.

But for real truth-telling they—both men and women—had to go online. Every time I blogged about the reticence problem, I was inundated with comments—almost a thousand altogether; once under the cover of anonymity, the real conversation began.

I was struck by how honest and helpful those comments were; when one raised a problem or a fear, others jumped in with solutions and encouragement. "Ladies, don't ever give up on this wonderful part of your life," wrote an enthusiast. "It's not just about the physical, it's about connecting with someone so deeply that it transcends all of our problems."

Many went out of their way to assure the rest that the point was not what you did but whether it reflected a sense of personal authenticity. "If you like sex, fantastic," wrote one, "and if you've had enough to last a lifetime and would rather have a foot rub—there's nothing wrong with you." And a number of men had words of reassurance for women who were self-conscious about their bodies. Some celebrated their partners—aging bodies and all. Others expressed gratitude for the acceptance they found, their own aging bodies and all.

Most of all, I was bowled over by the sheer number of people who defied my assumption—that we are embarrassed by the topic of sex—with their willingness to share their own experience and expertise online. One addressed a common problem this way: "Hope folks can handle the truth because there is no fun in painful sex. Don't pretend it doesn't hurt, because it doesn't have to." Another recurring issue was erectile dysfunction. "Being there myself, I recognize that Old Guy performance anxiety can impair one's partner's enjoyment," wrote another. He recommended Viagra.

There were even some sharp exchanges. When one woman wrote that in her experience "all sexual interest dried up after menopause, and that was such a relief. That energy is now diverted into activities in the community," another countered: "Speaking as an old lady who runs a charity, I think that community service and sexuality are not mutually exclusive." And some offered words of wisdom. "Sex is physics; love is chemistry."

Several comments expressed gratitude for access—at last!—to an honest discussion. "I've been stressing out about these issues recently, so it's wonderful to read such positive

comments," wrote one. Another thought honesty on the subject was overrated. "While my group of female friends has
always talked at length about many things, speaking graphically about their sex lives has not been one of them. Seems
tacky." Both comments confirmed that most people weren't
comfortable talking about sex face-to-face with anyone.

I think the recent popularity of the erotic novel *50 Shades
of Grey* is a dramatic example of the distance between the
graphic exuberance of the anonymous comments and the
shyness when women tried to raise the subject among themselves. Like the other bestsellers in the romance ($1.4 billion)
category, it is a bodice-ripper. It plays out the fantasy of being
seduced by a godlike suitor who desires us madly, beyond
anything he has ever known—a definite turn-on. (What goes
on in his "Red Room of Pain" is more a matter of taste.)

It has become a hit by word of mouth. Why are women my
age—including many of my friends—not only reading this
highly erotic and graphic series but talking about it? Given
what I have learned about the sexual circumstance of women
my age, I would suggest that we are reading it because
whether or not we are currently in a sexual relationship, we
want to confirm that our juices are still flowing. There is
enough unbonded—"pure vanilla," Grey calls it—eroticism in
the book to do that.

By talking about the book, we are also able to gauge
whether other women are exploring the same territory. "I'm

reading *50 Shades of Grey*" can be code for "I still have sexual feelings; do you?" When I mentioned the book in women's groups, there would be a rustle of interest; when I asked how many had read it or were planning to, I got a sea of hands. Once the conversation got going, many expressed the wish that they could talk more freely with their partners and share this part of their lives with close friends. "Having said that," one added, "I still don't know where to begin."

Maybe the place to begin is with the challenging statement I received in response to a recent blog on the subject:

> People under 50 don't talk about sex much either; they say only what is socially acceptable in their circle of friends and what they believe the others want to hear.
>
> We all have sexual desires we "shouldn't" have.
>
> We are all judgmental of the sexual behavior of others.
>
> We all tend to question our own sexuality.
>
> We all hold views and beliefs about sex that are strongly abhorred by others.
>
> Sexuality = vulnerability.
>
> Is it any wonder, then, that we are reluctant to discuss it socially except on the most superficial basis?

When I shared my "what's going on?" mission with my friend Laura Carstensen, who runs the Stanford Center on

Longevity, she was intrigued. The thing is, she mused, sex performed by aging bodies is as taboo a subject as aging itself. Even among those who study our behavior. Of all the studies she has supervised that show the older we get, the happier we get, none of them queried the respondents about their sex lives. Perhaps the researchers didn't know to look for sexual happiness, because they, like most of us, had not expected it to be a major source of joy at this stage of life.

One reason we don't talk about these things among ourselves, Carstensen suggests, is that as we move through the Second Adulthood years, there are more and more things that can go wrong. While we want to celebrate the good times and go after all that our reinvented lives have to offer, we are always aware of the disasters that lurk behind the same experiences. That lurking fatalism pervades our responses to even the most joyous and fulfilling events. It shapes our understanding of what it means to get older. At the same time, the awareness of interplay between the good stuff and the bad stuff makes us better able to focus on what's important and let go of lesser annoyances. Increasingly with age we learn to cherish what is.

In fact, one of the comments said as much. "One of the reasons that people might be satisfied with their sex lives as they age is that they finally learn to expect less and appreciate more. Lord knows, there is more and more that you can do nothing to change as you age." This tendency to appreciate the glass half full is, I have found, one of the gifts of this stage of life. It fosters a kind of emotional equilibrium that enables us to handle the chaotic nature of personal discovery— the mix of delight and bewilderment, curiosity and shame, satisfaction and guilt, success and failure.

The reason we need to talk about sex is not because we aren't talking about sex but because being forthcoming about what's going on in our new lives helps us better understand ourselves and each other. The lifetime of experience we thought we could count on can't answer the new questions we are asking. There is a lot to sort out. We are struggling with outgrown expectations for ourselves—we are not, as I keep saying, who we were, only older—and unmitigating prejudices against aging, so it is hard to get to an authentic statement of personal purpose. At the same time, the prospects for people our age of fulfillment, self-discovery, and making a difference are real. No wonder we often feel lost in a sea of unknowingness. Depending on the cards we are dealt in terms of health, finances, and life experience, how we play the hand of opportunities and limitations is the challenge of Second Adulthood.

"Don't fear change," reads a recent Facebook post. "Change fear." Easier said than done. I am inspired by the stories of women who have literally rewritten their life scripts. Often they can't explain how they did it; they just kept going, guided by their own internal lights and supported by the people who love them. I marvel at the determination and courage it takes to devote years to retraining themselves, or building a whole new business, or gearing up for a move across the country, or rebuilding their lives by sheer willpower after widowhood or divorce. Or simply daring to go for her personal "it."

No one ever said that reinvention would be easy. If it gets confusing at times, that is only because the territory is unfamiliar. The conversation about sex that I hope we will bring home from cyberspace can break through one more taboo that is blocking our way forward. The energy of sexuality, like the self-confidence of authenticity and the joy of discovery, is an expression of a rekindled spirit.

Chapter 1

Let Me Count the Ways

A recent study of brain scans found that love spurs the body to produce dopamine, a natural stimulant. "This activity was the same whether the individual was 18 or 50-plus. The body gets older but the basic emotion—the need to be in love—remains the same."

—Helen Fisher, *The First Sex*

Being in love knows no age limits. The kinds of love we can experience in a lifetime are limited only by our imagination and our circumstances. Every love, whenever and however often it strikes, is unique and mysterious. Yet for too many women the notion of experiencing that unique and mysterious intimacy at midlife seems preposterous; they have bought into the conventional wisdom that menopause is the last stop on the road to loneliness and decline.

An increasing number of other women know different; they are living—and defining—a totally new love narrative that is something fresh and surprising. At the same time that her aging body is continuing its lifelong production of dopamine, the hormonal reward of feeling love, a woman in this convention-defying group is experiencing love in ways she could not or would not have done earlier in her life. Her wants and needs are different, and she is fulfilling those unfamiliar desires—in both flesh and spirit. Not only are women still lusting and loving as they age, they are enjoying it more than ever.

Love is never easy, and each stage of life brings its own versions of heartbreak and ecstasy. The landscape of love we are entering at midlife is not without stumbling blocks and dark shadows. We all see long-term relationships foundering around us and widows who are lost and alone for the first time in decades. We know and certainly hear all too much about how hard it is for older women to find companionship, sex, respect. What we don't know enough about is how good love is for those who *are* enjoying it. This may be because the women who are revitalizing a long-standing relationship or finding a new one are afraid of jinxing the miracle by talking about it, or they may be afraid to "gloat" when their friends are complaining of loneliness and anemic sex lives.

If conventional wisdom focused less on loneliness and reflected more on how love is pursued, found, and sustained by women fifty and beyond, it would tell an entirely different story. We would learn that the universe of loving experiences includes a wider range of potential intimates than it did before, even though the absolute number may be more limited. We would learn that what we call love in our fifties, sixties, and seventies is not as narrowly defined as it was at earlier stages. Nor is it as single-minded and all-consuming. Many women don't even realize how widely and deeply they are experiencing love until they take inventory of the intimate connections that are enriching their lives now. So the first thing to ask ourselves and each other is how these new kinds of love—loves, really—feel.

There are many people to whom I regularly say "I love you"—and mean it—but as my outlook, priorities, and relationships have been reconsidered in recent years, I have noticed that in each case the feeling has recalibrated. I love my husband with more tolerance. I love my children with less need to make everything work out for them. I love my mother with more understanding. I love my friends with more—*everything,* especially trust and gratitude. And, oh, yes, I love me—sort of; which is to say I give myself a little more appreciation and a lot more slack. I *don't* love everyone in the whole world, nor do I want to be loved by all of them.

Most of my friends are in slightly different love constellations from mine. Many of them have never been married; others are divorced or widowed; some have children. And one friend has just fallen in love for the first time in her life—at sixty. We compare notes about autonomy and privacy and managing our lives and wonder what each of us is holding back. We can't quite imagine how love is for one another, yet as mysterious as our love trajectories appear to be, and as diverse as they look from the outside, my friends and I and other women I meet sense that something is going on in the way we experience intimacy these days. "Something going on" is a wake-up phrase for me. Everything I have learned about women—and about myself—started with a feeling of restless confusion. What's going on? Am I crazy? Am I the only one who feels this way?

I know one thing for sure—we are continuing to invent our lives as we go along. We are rewriting the rules of the game, including the game of love. No other generation of women has had such an open field to play in—the prospect of more healthy years ahead than our mothers and grandmothers. Moreover, those additional years are a midlife gift, not an add-on at the end. Laura Carstensen of the Stanford Center on Longevity suggests that it is more accurate to see the newfound block of time coming at the middle—from roughly age fifty to age seventy-five. That is the dynamic, rich, and rewarding stage I call Second Adulthood. It is a time of self-discovery and adventure as well as confusion and fear, but as we review and revise the many aspects of our lives, we find that, among other things we are capable of now, we are finally old enough to know what love is—or can be.

One important change as we age is that we have discarded the cultural delusions that often set our youthful selves off in the wrong direction. For too long, we pursued the holy grail of being "in love," and neglected the much more challenging and precious—and personally rewarding—work of "loving." This "dazzling vote of confidence for form over substance," write the authors of *A General Theory of Love*, gives short shrift to the kind of intimacy that can develop only from "the prolonged and detailed surveillance of a foreign soil."

The kind of intimacy—the New Intimacy—women are experiencing now is most definitely about loving. It involves vulnerability and boundaries. It always involves trust, and sometimes lust. Camaraderie and humor play a part. Empathy is essential, as are acceptance and respect. Shared experiences and values are more important than we might think. Chemistry doesn't disappear with maturity, it takes on more forms—a sexual tingle at the sight of an attractive person or the "click" when two people meet and know they are going to have lots to talk about or the blinding adoration for a grandchild. Friendship, physical appeal, and tenderness all constitute loving in the context I am writing about. The amalgam of these components is unique to each relationship a woman forms, as is the array of loving connections she assembles in her life. Each woman makes choices based on her evolving expectations and what her available options are. She may find intimacy without love (on the Internet, among other new locales). She may experience love without sex and sex without love. She may discover pure and simple love (with a child). And she may enjoy a love that is not related to a particular human being (for her work). All of the infinite variations can be satisfying, depending on the woman, her circumstances, and whether she is ready to move off the well-worn paths that have taken her this far. Those paths were carved by another woman—familiar but no longer defining. The most liberating insight of Second Adulthood is that You Are Not Who You Were, Only Older. And when we apply that prism to the landscape of love ahead, we can discover that there are so many more options than we might have expected.

WHAT IS IT LIKE TO BE IN LOVE NOW?

Women I meet are anxious to talk about how unexpected their experiences are. Much of what they tell me begins with an astonished "I can't believe that I am telling you this . . ." or "I can't believe I am doing this . . ." Their stories have helped me frame the issues I need to explore in order to understand what is going on. Every story has its own plotline, but overall they fall into very broad groupings. Some women are convinced that what they are finding is the Real Thing—at last. Others marvel in the rediscovery and revaluing of what has been there all along. Some are reveling in the freedom built into their new relationships, or the independence of "no strings attached." A number of women are especially gratified to discover new dimensions to their own capacity for love. And many are finding that their lives are enriched by commitments to people and projects that, although they may not get the dopamine flowing, feel very good indeed. Every one of them is exploring unknown territory, and all too many feel that they are lost, or alone. My goal in this book is to map that territory, together.

The anecdotes women have shared with me raise intriguing questions about the New Intimacy:

"I have fallen in love—with a short, balding, and very shy guy," a fifty-two-year-old bride tells me with a tinge of disbelief. Another admits, "I don't mind the way I would have in the past that he has only a GED while I have two master's degrees; he has a Ph.D. in life experience." Would they have fallen for the same guys thirty years ago, or would both have dismissed them as uncool or inappropriate, I wonder. Why now?

"All the things you worry about when you haven't dated as long as I hadn't dated—about sexual intimacy, about being attractive—none of that happened. Your body just kind of takes over," Martha told me in wonderment. "I was so comfortable and familiar with him. He made me feel like he really knew who I was—there was none of the 'Oh, my god, when he finds out about me . . .'—and I really knew who he was." How do we come to "know" each other after so much living? How does truth telling fit into loving? And self-knowledge?

"I have fallen in love with my husband all over again," exults a woman who has been married for decades. "There were times when I thought we would never make it, but this was worth hanging in for!" Other long-married couples like each other just fine, but, as one woman told me, "Our ther-mostats are at different levels." They treasure the history and the companionship they share and stay out of each other's way. What happens in a long-term relationship that refires the engine? Or sets it on neutral?

Then there are the women who have found that compan-ionship without sex or sex without commitment works for them, what one called a "no-stress hookup." They pal around with someone who probably wouldn't be a satisfactory full- time partner but is fun to travel with and is on a compat-ible wavelength. As a widely practiced form of intimacy, what does "companionship" mean for the near and the long haul?

Others are discovering that love has taken them in a totally unexpected direction. "I was happily married for forty years," says one woman, "but when my husband died, I found myself becoming increasingly drawn to other women. I just found the intimacy so easy." What is it like to make this kind of transfer of eroticism and intimacy? And what is it like for the women who never felt satisfied in their heterosexual relationships who are discovering their true sexuality now?

"You may be shocked," says a very serious-looking doctor, "but I have discovered the joys of one-night stands. I need a rest from 'relating.' And the sex is great!" I am not shocked; I have spoken to countless women who are experimenting with separating sex from commitment, and even a few who have discovered that they are "polyamorous" and are adding additional players to their primary relationships; others have found that "married dating" Web sites ("four million bozos and a small collection of well-intended, articulate males," one woman told me) offer another kind of intimacy. Does the release of our inner troublemaker in what I call the Fuck-You Fifties set us free to literally go anywhere?

When talking about love, women—regardless of the status of their other relationships—include deepening devotion to their women friends. They are exhilarated by new levels of understanding and trust that surpass all other connections in their lives. What is it like to build on a long-standing friendship? What is it like to fall out of love with an old friend? To make a new friend?

Women have not been generating such questions until now. In order to answer them and to illuminate this unprecedented experience—to figure out what's going on—I framed my own set of questions.

I began conducting long interviews with a wide range of women (and some men), and I also posted a questionnaire on several Web sites I count on for open, honest, and safe conversation (see Resources list). Here is what I asked:

Are you in love now? If so, does it feel different from other times in your life? How? Is your partner someone you would have picked (or did pick) back then? Or someone totally different?

If not, would you say you were "in sex"? (Meaning enjoying sex even though the relationship couldn't be called love. If so, is there anything new about the sex?)

Have you found out anything about the way you love now? Are you less/more interested in companionship and doing things together? Are you less/more interested in monogamy? (Or are you a "serial monogamist"?)

If you are aware of power differentials or abuses of power in previous relationships, can you describe them and whether things are different now?

If you are not in love now and wish you were, what is it you miss?

If you are not in love now and like that just fine, what do you like about your situation?

Are you feeling what you used to call "love" for people in your life who aren't romantic or sexual partners? (Friends or grandchildren, for example.)

The answers came pouring in. I am sure that many of the women who didn't answer felt so out of the game, they had nothing to say about love, and that others were so unhappy, they couldn't talk about it. So I assume that my respondents were, in general, more upbeat than the statistical proportion of women in their fifties, sixties, and seventies. But because what I was looking for was information about the experiences of women who were in love or had a clear idea of how love would be different for them now, the self-selected responses tell the story. Some were long and detailed, tracing lives of love and loss and reinvention. Others described discoveries about themselves and challenges to rules that no longer make sense. "After having been married and divorced twice and raising a daughter mostly on my own," one woman wrote, "I've come to realize I'm more comfortable as a 'serial monogamist.'" Her current "soul mate" lives in a different state. "I enjoy running my own life, on my schedule," she says, "and when we get together, it's like a holiday that never ends! It's time we broke out of the married-or-single mind-set to realize that there are all kinds of relationships in between."

Other responses were short and poignant, like this e-mail from Mindy: "I will be fifty in a few weeks, if I live that long. I am dying of colon cancer at the moment. I live with the love of my life in northern California, and I have never been happier in my life. I have three grown children and seven grandchildren, with another due soon. I am having the best sex I have ever had in my life too—even though I am this sick. It's like I am using his energy and I don't have to expend any of my own."

Still others reflected a personal journey. "I haven't been 'in love' for more than ten years," one wrote. "At first, it was a choice. I thought it was high time I examined why I kept falling in love with the 'same guy' (as in 'same guy, different penis'). A year turned into two . . . and then ten. Mostly, I think, because it took me that long to get clear on who I am and why those men held such fascination for me. Now when I consider the prospect of being in love, I am most intrigued by the possibility that I could actually be who I am . . . with someone who gets me."

Janet was less optimistic; she was still mourning a faded fairy tale. "Those of us who are desperate for love and attention—to what lengths do or will we go to find that? Believing in what we are told—are we so naïve—so much in need to believe in movies like *Pretty Woman* and those stories of knights coming to rescue us from harm and sweep us off our feet? Can we have our cake and eat it too? I used to think so, but now, after all these years, I say no."

Many described evolving relationships. "Our love has mellowed into a deep bond of friendship and shared life experiences," writes Della about her long marriage. "Yes, romance is still there. But the relationship is not rife with the up-and-down mix of emotions there was in the beginning of our marriage. Rather, there's trust, safety, love, and mutual support that only the years can bring."

When I interviewed women in person there was another element in the conversation—what I came to recognize as the "eyes-light-up" factor; that is, the delight with which they talked about a special person—a partner, a grandchild, a friend, a special student, frequently (especially mothers who have sons only) a daughter-in-law. This expression of comfort and joy is not only metaphorical; the glow is due to a literal shot of hormonal delight that nature has granted us throughout our lives. Countless studies show that in moments of intimacy, oxytocin—the so-called "cuddle" or "social bonding" hormone—is released into the bloodstream. The first bond is the gaze between mother and child, but others accumulate throughout our lives with every trusting and tender relationship we establish.

As those eyes-light-up conversations got going, we compared notes and found we shared many insights: We are more confident about being able to count on those we love than before. We feel more intensely about the inner orbit of our constellation of intimates and less about the people we are shifting to the outer rings. We are clearer about what we expect from those we love and more accepting of what isn't going to happen. We accept and sometimes cherish the places where love of another cannot go—that inner sanctum where each of us is on her own.

HOW "GIVE" AND "TAKE" HAVE CHANGED

These shifts in our perceptions have a lot to do with who the woman doing the loving is now. As diverse as the expressions of love are, they have certain newly acquired psychological characteristics in common. For one thing, they reflect a sense of confidence that has been unfamiliar to most of us in decades past. At last we know who we are—and who we aren't; we know what the world is like, which makes it easier to know what is possible and go for it. At the same time, our expectations are more realistic than back when love was what dreams were made of. We don't try to change anyone (very much) and we don't look for a perfect fit or a protector. To whatever degree we are financially secure—a major and immensely stressful consideration in Second Adulthood—we are definitely better at managing on our own, not sweating the small stuff, and living with the insecurity of ongoing change.

How women get to this state of mind is the collective story of each individual reinvention. I have spent most of my professional life chronicling that transformation of women's lives at different stages, and the experience has, in turn, inspired and empowered my own. Every time over the past forty years that I posed the question "What's going on with women?" the answers were different. I first became curious about something going on back in the seventies when I was editor of *Ms.* magazine. Our readers were high school students and grandmothers, homemakers and rebels, but if there was one driving editorial principle behind that breakthrough journalistic adventure, it was that if one woman was experiencing something, it was certain that other women were too, only they were not talking about it; the magazine needed to tell such stories and open up the conversation. To do that we needed a vocabulary to describe the heretofore "unspeakable" or unspoken of. Back then it was such experiences as "sexual harassment" and "reproductive freedom" that were being named and brought into light. Having the vocabulary was essential to sharing our experiences and galvanizing a force for change. We need to do so again. We haven't yet found the words to demystify (another important term) all that we are feeling in Second Adulthood.

When in my early fifties I began to feel dissatisfied and restless, that faith in shared experience led me to suspect that there was something going on. I checked it out with other women, and sure enough, they felt it too. *Inventing the Rest of Our Lives: Women in Second Adulthood* was the result of my search for understanding and reassurance that I wasn't crazy—or under some menopausal spell—and that neither were the hundreds of women I talked to. (I have always loved a T-shirt I saw once that said "This is not a hot flash. It's a power surge.") After that book came out, other women who were in the process of navigating that transition came forward and, building on the language I had offered to describe our shared experience, we could talk with more clarity. The more we shared, the more I began to see some guiding insights that would be helpful to anyone negotiating the bumpy road to the new stage of life. *Fifty Is the New Fifty: Ten Life Lessons for Women in Second Adulthood* was my effort to interpret their discoveries and disappointments. This book is a deeper exploration of the new stage of life we are defining as we go along through the all-important lens of love.

That new stage of life is characterized by questions, doubts, and bewilderment and also by daring, discovery, and redefinition. The years around fifty and beyond are "about redefining their choices, whether that be their career, their marriage, or their friendships, and asking themselves key questions about whether or not they are living authentically," a woman who works with midlife professional women wrote me. "Obviously," she went on with insight and clarity, "there will be sadness and a feeling of loss as women go through this assessment and reevaluation process, but for most of the women I work with, once they have come through the other side of that process, they are invigorated, reborn, and passionate about what this next stage of their lives will bring."

Dealing with all that confusion and change forces us to mobilize our resources—for courage, for self-discovery, for coping with insecurity. Every time we recalibrate some part of ourselves, we have to handle the upheaval that change engenders. To understand the magnitude of this upheaval, we have only to look back on our first major life transition—adolescence. Wildly fluctuating hormones are not the only similarity. Now, as then, we are asking ourselves questions: about ourselves—"who am I?"; about the future—"what do I want to do with my life?"; and about relationships—"who will I love? How will I love them?" For many, the most invigorating symptom of this second transition is an almost adolescent defiance that washes over us as our estrogen retreats. There comes a day for each of us when we blurt out the startling revelation "I don't care what people think anymore!" That phrase becomes the rallying cry of the Fuck-You Fifties. After a lifetime of seeking approval, the notion of rejecting it is mind-blowing. Sex may be the first frontier a midlife woman crosses or the last, but "crossing the line" is what sets us on new paths. "If women are having sex because they want to," observe the authors of *Still Doing It: The Intimate Lives of*

Women over Sixty, "what other desires might they pursue in every aspect of their lives?"

At the same time, we are afraid. Afraid of failing, of being rejected, of being ridiculous or pitiful. Intimacy at any point in life is about the risk of becoming vulnerable to another person, trusting another person. When you combine those fears with that of exposing a battered and bruised heart and a no-less-beat-up body to a "stranger," it is no wonder that the prospect looks doubtful.

"Intimacy is the opposite of fear," one woman told me as she described her newfound outlook. "I want to love because I choose to love, not because I feel I have no other options. I find 'heat' relationships easy, but shallow, though I enjoy the sexual passion that results from fantasies of who that person is. To move beyond one's fears of intimacy and truth with another person takes an incredible amount of courage. I think the inability to work through difficulties in a relationship to build true intimacy is what kills sexual passion. I want to believe that two people can work through their issues and ultimately find real intimacy through acceptance of each other as people and thus create a place of safety for each other."

Where does that kind of courage come from? From asking yourself tough questions and not finding the answers you expected. From making a fool of yourself while trying out new behaviors. From coping with life as it is. And getting to know yourself for real. A tall order, not to be filled by a weekend at a spa. In most of the conversations about self-discovery, the notion of a real time-out—a period of self-reflection and doubt—comes up. A serious pause to regroup while the atoms of our lives are shifting. The pause can go on for a year or two of floating aimlessly (but not really) in what I call the Fertile Void. The irony of those words is intentional. In so many situations our uncharacteristic behavior is dismissed as fallout from the loss of biological fertility our hormones are dealing with; I have found that, to the contrary, we are going through a confusing but creative period of great emotional, professional, and psychological fertility, but only if we give ourselves the time and the slack we need to figure things out.

The first reaction to this unfamiliar state of mind is a panicky scramble to manage the outcome of events that seem to be spinning out of control. When, despite our best efforts, we can't come up with answers and solutions, it is easy to blame ourselves for being indecisive, ineffective, even—buying into the cultural disdain—"hormonal." Some women discount their own feelings of curiosity and discomfort and get so caught up in their menopausal symptoms that they ignore the signs of an emerging self. Uncomfortable as it is, though, not knowing what's happening makes room for the unexpected to happen and for fresh ways of responding to our circumstances to emerge. During that time-out we begin to explore our notions of intimacy and to reconsider established relationships. Out of confusion comes insight, as Mary's account suggests.

"I'm just about to turn fifty," she began. "I've been struggling with very painful feelings of 'What next?' 'What does my life mean?' 'Is my relationship with my husband still the be-all and end-all of my life (as it used to be)?' In my heart I know the answer to the last question—I wanted, and still want, the man that I married almost thirty years ago to be in my life, but he can no longer be at the center of it. This realization came with overwhelming feelings of guilt, bewilderment, and anguish.

"I also felt totally disillusioned with my career of teaching, realizing that I had been struggling with it for a long time and needed a change. . . .

"I kept on fighting the feelings of dissatisfaction and anxiety till I was almost on the verge of a breakdown. Finally I acknowledged that I had to get away for a while and took off to New Zealand for seven weeks. In many ways a life-changing experience, primarily because I met so many wonderful people, but also because I began to lose that 'neediness' which was always nagging away at me—I came to appreciate my own company and the fact that not everyone I met would want to engage with me.

"However, on returning home my feelings of 'stuckness' and fear also returned, especially in relationship to my marriage. . . . But now for the first time in a long time I feel 'still' and able to make choices on my terms—if I stay with my husband it will be because I want to, not because I have to, through fear of the unknown. I may never write that great novel or save the world but I am beginning to relish the small things I can do and I'm looking forward to the next stage of my life. . . . I know I will travel more, perhaps go abroad to do voluntary work, work on my language skills, write, and keep in touch with the new acquaintances I met in NZ."

During the time Mary wandered in the Fertile Void, the need to recalibrate her marriage receded as a priority behind getting her self "unstuck." In the meantime, she is finding that, unexpectedly, the major new source of nourishment and power is not in rekindled romance but in independence and outreach.

Similarly, in Gerry's reconsideration of her life, the internal process has become the reward, regardless of the consequences. "Before I began to question and ask the questions that weren't allowed to be asked, I felt like I was dying inside," she says. Today she is energized, if terrified. "I like that I am pushing myself to be truthful. To face up to all of the things that I have hidden from myself and been afraid to face. It's liberating to speak the truth. So, though it's a scary process and my marriage is in a crisis mode, I can't see how I can lose in this process. I am growing and I am learning."

WHAT WE KNOW ABOUT OURSELVES

We each pass through the miasma of unknowing in our own way, but there are also some guideposts to the journey toward a New Intimacy. I identified ten in my last book, but I have singled out the most relevant, and redefined each one as it pertains to what we are talking about here.

You Are Not Who You Were, Only Older. Neither are your relationships.

All of the confidence and daring that we are accumulating, all the questions we are asking, change our perspective on love. Even if the partner stays the same, the dynamic changes. "Marriage is a game for adult players," Robertson Davies wrote in *The Lyre of Orpheus*, "and the rules in every marriage are different." More important, the women I have interviewed would add, the rules are also "different at every stage of the marriage."

No **Is Not a Four-Letter Word.** The major breakthrough to Second Adulthood is learning to exercise the power of *no*. When you look back on all the *yes*es you expended on being liked, being approved of, being loved (and the one big *no* you were trained to save for sex), you can see how apocalyptic reversing the ratio can be. A further refinement—**Saying No 2.0**—is learning to say no without giving an excuse or explanation; the fact that you don't want to do it is enough. Popular relationship adviser Byron Katie puts the no/yes equation into a pertinent context in *I Need Your Love—Is That True?*:

"My lover is the place inside me where an honest yes or no comes from. That's my true partner. It's always there. And to tell you yes when my integrity says no is to divorce that partner." In the creation of an intimate relationship, that inner power translates into authoritative expressions of will and the assertion of long-neglected demands of our own.

A corollary of that assertion of personal authority is the recognition that it is about time we **Do Unto Ourselves as We Have Been Doing Unto Others.** This doesn't mean abandoning caring, generous, forgiving, and empathetic impulses that are what love is about; it is just sending some of that acceptance and nurturing back in our own direction. In her book *A Long Bright Future*, gerontologist Carstensen describes a psychological equipoise that enhances a new kind of loving care. This is a time, she writes, "when cognition and emotion blend optimally in ways that give people insights into themselves and others." Or, as another woman told me when I asked if her experience of love had changed, "I love more deeply—and with less judgment."

No small factor in this more balanced kind of intimacy is, for many of us, the absence of our children. The much-bemoaned empty nest has removed the intensity of attending to them and sacrificing for them; it has also given many women the chance to feather their own nests with plans and experiences. For those embarking on new relationships, not having to take into account their own parenting demands and responsibilities or evaluate a prospective partner's parenting skills expands their horizons dramatically.

Both/And* Is the New *Either/Or. In the process of loving "more deeply and with less judgment," we find ourselves discarding either/or standards that guided earlier interpersonal behavior: whether a prospective partner was Mr. Right or Mr. Wrong, whether a gut feeling about someone was smart or dumb, whether a crisis was the be-all or the end-all, whether to be guided by your biological clock or your heart. Choices are not so clear-cut and definitive anymore; options look more nuanced, relationships seem less fraught. As many gerontologists have observed, age brings a noticeable "mellowness." We can take the bad that besets us with the good that we may have undervalued. The glass looks half full as often as it does half empty. As we evaluate our relationships—old or new—that is a particularly crucial change of perspective.

Our changing understanding of intimacy only reinforces the essential truism of life, love, and survival in Second Adulthood: **A "Circle of Trust" Is a Must.** For many women, these are the most intimate, trusting, enjoyable relationships of all. Friendships are the gold standard for love as we are redefining it. Even for those whose most all-consuming passion lies elsewhere, friends, they acknowledge, make it all possible. In the movie *It's Complicated*—directed by a woman of a certain age, Nancy Meyers—about a woman whose ex-husband is trying to woo her back, Meryl Streep's character is energized by evenings in the freewheeling and hilarious company of her girlfriends. They can't *believe* some of the choices she is making, but they are with her 100 percent. In her book, Jenny Sanford, the wife of the South Carolina governor who, it was revealed, was regularly running down to Buenos Aires to see another woman, says she could never have coped without the support and loyalty she got from her circle of trust; they couldn't *believe* he could be such a jerk!

Armed with refreshed self-awareness and mastery—and a trusted posse watching our backs—we are redefining the quest for love and the practice of intimacy. Whether it is a no-future sexual escapade or a rediscovered partner from the past, an Internet adventure or a revitalized long-term marriage, women in love are establishing models of trust and caring that are fresh and strong. Speaking truth, and especially speaking truth to power, becomes the currency, and discovering the truth about ourselves—authenticity—becomes a goal. Not the classic ingredients of a love story. We are writing a whole new tale.

In the following chapters, I will try to tell that new love story: Why love feels different now. How it is different. How *we* are different—in body, mind, and spirit. And how this New

Intimacy affects the choices we make as we reinvent the rest of our lives. That story is really many stories—of bewilderment, fear, discovery, heartbreak, and joy. By gathering and interpreting them here, I hope we will all be better able to understand and celebrate *what's going on*.

CHAPTER 2

"Interdependence" and the New Intimacy

> Romantic love is the story of how you need another
> person to complete you. It is an absolutely insane story.
> My experience is that I need no one to complete me.
> As soon as I realize that, everyone completes me.
>
> — Byron Katie, *I Need Your Love—Is That True?*

Intimacy is a contract we enter into with another person. It can be a lifelong commitment or just a handshake, but for it to bind, both parties need to sign on to the terms. Until recently, though, the terms were rarely fair to both parties, because they were based on power, not commitment.

Historically, intimacy has been accompanied by insecurity and fear, because it has been regulated by the one (almost always male) who controlled the money, who had more professional or social status, who fought more forcefully, whose approval mattered more, who protected whom, who couldn't leave. Abuses of such power caused much suffering. And many of the women you will meet in this book know about those abuses firsthand. For them it is essential to anticipate the practical pitfalls—with prenuptial agreements and health proxies, for example—and to be alert to the choices that can lead to power plays and resentments—avoiding a joined-at-the-hip social life, designing workable financial arrangements, managing family obligations. That wariness about giving away the store combined with the emergence of women of our generation who have more control over their own store make for more realistic and achievable expectations. At the same time, we have learned a thing or two about another aspect of power—the power to change another person to fill a need or desire. Most valuable, we have learned the importance of empowering ourselves rather than waiting to be rescued from our own lives.

As varied as our circumstances may be, we can learn from one another about establishing parameters and letting go. Long-married couples can tell us about learning to cherish the familiar and explore the unknown. The sexually timid women who are discovering the joys of sex—with women as well as men—embody the freedom that comes with Second Adulthood. The widows who are incorporating the best of a past marriage into a new one have much to say about sharing the second half of life. Divorced women taking a second chance on love offer a very practical view of how to establish emotional, social, and financial boundaries. Those committed to single life are defining a meaningful and chosen lifestyle; they are finding the love they want—reliability without responsibility, for example, or simply some peace and quiet—while also enjoying their freedom. The experienced daters are learning to tell the difference between a potential partner and a man who is looking for only "a nurse with a purse." What their discoveries have in common is that they are about what a woman wants, not what she "needs."

Not that need has no place in the equation. We all require a certain mix of strengths, virtues, and chemistry in order to connect with another person and thrive in their company. The big change, though, is that those needs have nothing to do with neediness. The joy of maturity lies in the fact that wants and needs can be expressions of self-esteem and individuality on the part of someone who can manage just fine if those wants and needs aren't forthcoming. Neediness is the plaintive and passive longing of someone waiting to be rescued.

This change of heart can be especially disruptive to a long-standing relationship in which dependency has become ingrained. The risks of challenging the benefactor figure in a marriage are enormous, but so are the rewards. For some women, making change leads to a new level of devotion mellowed by years of discovery and disappointment; for others, reinventing intimacy reveals resources of forthrightness and courage in both partners; others may establish new terms of individual empowerment and mutual support. "When we finally learned to 'raise our tolerances and lower our expectations,' as a therapist had suggested, things began to improve," Becky wrote me. "We began to accept the reality of who we are rather than the expectation of who we thought the other should be."

This kind of accommodation is not about compromising expectations; it is about establishing expectations on a bedrock of acceptance that can support them. Even women who aren't currently in love with a partner sense the shift too. Many of them tell me that they would now enter an intimate relationship from a new baseline of self-sufficiency and curiosity. In a panel discussion about my last book, *Fifty Is the New Fifty*, Gloria Steinem, who is seventy-five, put it this way: "The biggest surprise for me is that you're not obsessed with sex anymore. And you don't experience that as a loss; it's not a loss; it's not better or worse; it's just different. I look at young couples in the street and I feel like that song from *The King and I*—'Hello, Young Lovers'—and I think, Oh, I remember that. There is no way that anybody could have told me in my younger years that this would not be a loss, but it's not. It's exactly as wonderful, but in a different way. . . . You are now free to be devoted to other things. Here's the key difference: When you have sex you enjoy it, but when you are not having sex you are not obsessed with it." Obsession is a neediness that no longer applies.

On the same panel Isabella Rossellini, who is fifty-seven, admitted that she had been what is often called "a man junkie." "I always thought when I was younger that I had to have a man, that I had to have a companion or a husband. So if a relationship came to an end, I was very busy looking for the other person. I don't know what I was thinking—that I couldn't be complete or that I would just go gray and fat and my life will come to an end . . . or the fear of going to the movies by myself, traveling by myself—it never occurred to me that that was a possibility. Then I went to a therapist. I told her that since I always had a boyfriend or a companion, one after the other, it's so hard for me to stay a week without one. She said, 'Try to be alone for six months'—as medicine she gave me that advice. And I loved it! To my surprise. Life became very quiet. I could concentrate. I could take care of the children. There were no conflicts. Obviously," she added, "if I fall in love or if I find a person, but that's a different story from seeking constantly companionship, a male companionship. If I fell in love now, I'd even get married, but now

I am not in love, so here I am making my films and raising my children." For her, the discovery is that not being in love doesn't mean not being fulfilled.

FULFILLMENT AND/OR LOVE

A sixty-seven-year-old woman who describes herself as "independent and generally interested in the world" wrote me that she is looking for a love partner, but she is also quite content with where her life is, which is a whole lot better than where it was. Her present life, she sums up "is fine compared to a tense relationship in which I didn't feel valued. I have had and continue to have an interesting life—anthropologist, Peace Corps, yoga teacher, lots of good stuff! But it would be better with a boyfriend." Or, in the words of a Holly Near song she likes to quote, "An old camp fire gets warmer with you around it, but even when you're gone, it still cooks the stew." Feeling valued, she has found, is an experience she can give herself.

Camille can most definitely do without. "Married twice. Probably won't do it again. Had many lovers. Currently live alone (with cat) and love it. Have a 'friend with benefits' and there's always the bedside toys when I don't want to be bothered with him."

WomanSage—a nationwide network of feisty women over forty-five—recently queried its married members; if their marriage ended, they were asked, would they want to remarry or establish a "committed relationship." As Jane Haas, the founder of the organization, reported, roughly the same number voted for marriage as for "living in sin"; the latter group included several who had spent years caretaking a sick husband and were determined not to play nurse again. But the big surprise was that the same number, one-third of the respondents, didn't want a serious relationship of any kind. That group was, Haas reports, for the most part, financially secure. "Women who work or who can support themselves tell me they want to make their own decisions after midlife."

Which is not to say they want to be taken for a ride. "I am not looking for a wealthy man," Lynn wrote me, "but it would be nice to find a man who at least could pay his way when we go out. Much less go on vacation sometimes, own his home, or even have a retirement plan. I have all these things," she goes on. "(And NO, I did not get any of them through divorce.)" Indeed, in every category, the New Intimacy is very much affected by financial considerations and values. Earning, allocating, and spending—and sharing—money is a big part of any emotional contract we make.

A group of financially self-sustaining women—one that is growing—is "still single." In a 2008 census, they represented 11 percent of women between the ages of forty-five and fifty-four. Some of them will ultimately pair up with someone, while others are becoming more and more committed to life on their own. They have work, friends, children of friends and siblings, online communities, and a freewheeling approach to opportunity. They also have romantic relationships. "I've learned something from every man I have dated; I don't have anything bad to say about them," one woman told *More* magazine. Another summed up her situation this way: "Marriage just isn't for me."

Phoebe, who is in her sixties, had built a rich and interesting life for herself that included good friends, interesting work, lots of travel, and some disappointing relationships. Marriage, it seemed, was not for her either. She had little to do with her blood family, but her "chosen family" embraced her as warmly as she could ever want; the love she gave and got from that carefully selected group created the most intimate resource in her adult life. When she met someone for whom she felt an even deeper love, Phoebe had no intention of choosing the intimacy between them over all others; she wanted to add him to that company. As a friend of mine described it, "The wedding took place in the beautiful home of Phoebe's close friends on a bluff overlooking the sea. Many of us flew in to be there. The bishop who married them was a close friend of hers; the groom's oldest friend read a poem and served as groomsman; Phoebe's goddaughter stood up for her. It was just a spectacular outpouring of love for the lovers." Neither of them felt that they needed to forsake all others to fulfill their commitment to each other.

WANTING BUT NOT NEEDING

Un-neediness is a very recent development in the creation of new love relationships; it is just as recent a development in many established ones.

Carrie's marriage, for example, evolved into a more equitable give-and-take. Looking back on the early years, she says, "In my forty-four-year relationship with my husband, we haven't so much had a shift in power, but we have had more of a division of power. More sharing the responsibility regardless of the nature of the particular duty over time." Whether they are starting over or renegotiating a long-term relationship, women are establishing a revised contract based not on power and control but on balance and cooperation. It is premised on the understanding that while each partner could make it emotionally and financially on their own, they want to pool their resources in a mutually defined version of equality.

Pooled resources are the opposite of a win-lose notion of power and compliance. Our newfound capability to stand up for ourselves—to speak truth to power—also makes it possible to negotiate compromise from a position of strength. We are simply tougher. Menopause cuts down the production of the hormones that, according to neuropsychiatrist Dr. Louann Brizendine, feed a woman's "communication circuits, emotion circuits, the drive to tend and care, and the urge to avoid conflict at all costs."

At the same time, we have moved beyond the more rigid outlook that put every conflict into an all-or-nothing show-down. Our acceptance of the imperfections in most things has created room for many more options. A later-life brain development fosters a more flexible response to life's challenges. In *The Mature Mind,* psychiatrist and gerontologist Gene D. Cohen describes changes in the brain that enhance the ability "to contemplate more than one answer to a problem, to consider contradictory solutions to life's challenges, and to recognize how much in life is relative." These, he maintains, "are exactly the tools we need" as we feel our way toward establishing balance in our relationships.

PLAYING BY THE ROLES

So much holds us back—history, tradition, and the old order, for starters. On top of that, there are real and acquired gender differences that make it harder to explain and understand each other. The degree to which gender roles get in the way of integrating thoughts and feelings, wants and needs, into a thriving relationship is suggested in a recent study of same-sex couples, where presumably the playing field was more equal. Of course, same-sex couples have their own problems with roles and power, but when it comes to knowing what the other person is really saying, they seem to have more understanding.

Several recent studies have shown that lesbian and gay part-
nerships are far more egalitarian overall than heterosexual ones;
household tasks were shared, and so was the willingness to
work on the relationship. In heterosexual couples, the old para-
digms still held—women did far more of the housework and
men were more likely to have the financial responsibility; men
were more likely to initiate sex and women were more likely
to initiate a conversation about problems in the relationship.

Here is how Amelia and Grace, two formerly married
women who fell in love when they were in their fifties,
describe the magic in their long-standing relationship in
Late-Life Love by Connie Goldman. "Although each of us has
her own strengths," says Amelia, "I feel equal when I'm with
Grace. Our days aren't fraught with agonizing thoughts,
such as 'Am I loved? Am I still loved? Are you going to leave
me?' We have a calm and steady relationship. It's the way that
it ought to be. You depend on each other, love and respect
each other. We spend most of our time together. Not many
days go by that we don't say, 'How lucky we are!' "

Equals even argue better, according to one study, because
each understands where the other is coming from. "The ability to see the other person's point of view appears to be more
automatic in same-sex couples," the researchers report, but
there is hope for heterosexuals. Those "who can relate to
their partner's concerns and who are skilled at defusing

arguments also have stronger relationships." I am reminded of a cartoon in which a couple is arguing fiercely, and the man is saying, "I'm not yelling at you, I'm yelling *with* you!"

The old differences still linger on the path to a New Intimacy, of course; the most deeply rooted are the different ways in which the genders experience closeness. Many popular books have pointed out that men feel connected when *doing* things side by side; women need to talk, even just casually, if we are to make contact. If serious conversation is involved, men are generally more comfortable looking straight ahead, as in driving; women crave eye contact. Luckily, such disconnects modify with age. As women become more independent and assertive—less needy—they have less need to establish "deep, intense, verbal connections with others," says biological anthropologist Helen Fisher. Men, on the other hand, seek out connection and tenderness as they age.

A psychiatrist who specializes in men at midlife confirms that pattern. Among his patients who are looking for something that is missing in their marriages or that they are hoping to find in a new relationship, he hears a longing for "someone who will listen, who will take an interest in them, who they can talk to," he says. "When there is trouble in a relationship they say they feel 'unappreciated.'" Sound familiar? When I asked him whether his patients wanted that kind of connection earlier in their lives, he looked at me and asked, "What do *you* think?" Fisher observes that "as male and female baby boomers reach middle age in many societies, their definitions of intimacy may converge. This may serve to strengthen" the equal footing in what some sociologists call "peer marriages."

POWER PLAYS

For women, a "peer" relationship means shedding feelings of powerlessness and accommodation; for men it means relinquishing some of the power they have been granted by virtue of being male. Paul, who is in his early fifties, is a not-there-yet man. He has what might be called a "peer divorce;" the day-to-day relationship with his two children is his first priority and primary source of joy. He and his ex-wife live in the same apartment building and the kids move from one apartment to the other during the week. "When they're not with me," he says, "I feel empty, even if I'm with someone." Which is not to say that he isn't looking for his next relationship. In fact, he has signed up with not one but two marriage brokers. He says he wants to meet independent women. "I used to be attracted to very needy broken-wing women who needed rescuing," he recalls. But no more; he has come to "understand the concept that a women could love me, but not really need me."

While he is into emotional equality, Paul is also strongly invested in perks from the past—particularly the powerful role of the more mature older man. "Somebody gave me this rule of thumb: a perfect age of the right woman is half the guy's age plus ten." That sounds good to him, but he breaks the pool of younger women down further in terms of the demands they make on him. "There's basically three different age groups that I have dated, and two out of the three worked for me and the third doesn't work and it doesn't work very quickly," he explains. "There's women, I would say, from twenty-eight to their early thirties; they're eligible for me because they're generally not thinking yet about having children—they're young and they still want to have fun. But they're kind of immature and they're always constantly texting. I feel like with those women I have to buy condoms for my BlackBerry; the BlackBerry gets more action than I do.

"Then there are women in their midthirties to early forties, and they've been married and have children—and they really have very good perspective, you know, they don't still have the fantasy marriage in their heads, their children are their priorities, they understand that my kids are my priorities, and that actually kind of works well. And then the women in the middle, like in their midthirties or forties that haven't been married and haven't had kids, they're completely insane. You sit down with them and within five or ten minutes they want to know how long you were married, where you live, where your ex-wife lives, how long you've been divorced, why you got divorced, how many kids you have, how often you see them, and if you want more children.

That's pretty much the date, and so it's kind of—they're on a real mission because their biological clock is going crazy."

Paul's mixed message—finding fulfillment in coparenting with his ex-wife and at the same time making age superiority a requirement in future relationships—illustrates the difficulty many contemporary men have in sharing power and making themselves vulnerable. Carol Gilligan, in her groundbreaking book *The Birth of Pleasure,* draws a connection between the two within a historic dynamic that affects both men and women, the powerful and the powerless. "Patriarchy drains pleasure because hierarchy leads us to cover vulnerability," she explains. Vulnerability is, of course, the essence of intimacy.

FROM DEPENDENCE TO INDEPENDENCE TO INTERDEPENDENCE

Bella Abzug, the feisty, fearless, and brilliant congresswoman and feminist, understood power, characteristically, in both its political and personal sense. Some considered her marriage a reversal of roles; she made news, while Martin, a stockbroker and novelist, was the go-to parent for their two daughters, but in reality they supported each other. Soon after Martin died, Bella tried to put the dynamic between them into words: "My reputation is that of an extremely independent woman, and I am. But I was dependent, clearly, on Martin. He would embrace me in his furry chest and warm heart and protect me from the meanness one experiences in the kind of life I lead."

In the politics of intimacy, Bella saw the progression from the needy and anxious-to-please model of prefeminist times to the present day, when a woman can make it on her own, as a revolution that took us from dependence to independence. But she also talked about a next and necessary revolution: creating a way of achieving intimacy through *inter*dependence. Not easily done. How do you come to know the distinction between vulnerability and neediness, between invulnerability and independence? The answers to those questions are both a challenge and a promise.

Interdependence does not require that every responsibility and emotional exchange is split down the middle—or that every responsibility and experience, even every expectation, is shared. Simply that the equation feels fair to both parties. And that the relationship is enriching to both. The poet Rainer Maria Rilke describes an intimacy "in which each partner appoints the other to be the guardian of his solitude, and thus they show each other the greatest possible trust." Or, as Gloria Steinem put it when she married for the first time at sixty-seven, "We wanted to be responsible for each other." Sadly, that mutual responsibility soon turned into six months of intensive caregiving as her husband of three years succumbed to a brain tumor. Women who find love at Steinem's age are well aware that time is not on their side. Yet most would say that the risk is well worth taking.

CALLING OUR OWN SHOTS

More than ever before in history a midlife woman is mistress of her own fate. How much so can be seen in two personal ads written about four decades apart. When we were in our twenties, a friend of mine and I—dismayed by the too-good-to-be-true notices we found in the *New York Review of Books*—decided to write a truly accurate description of our situation. The one we composed, with tongue only partially in cheek, went like this: "Fat, uptight wallflower, approaching her prime, seeks Heathcliff." Contrast our haikulike testament to insecurity with this particularly detailed ad in a recent issue of an Ivy League alumni magazine:

> **Bright, captivating,** affectionate artist and outdoor adventurer. Graceful, natural athlete, leggy slim figure, easygoing great looks, 49. International experience and sophistication yet deep roots in New England with the best of its philosophy and love of its landscape and light. Mischievous and genuine, sexy and comfortable with herself. Loves challenge of the elements: downhill skiing, sailing, hiking, breathtaking views. Passionate about photography, architecture, Maine,

Japan (spent 3 years there), spur of the moment fun, the environment. Authentic, game. Contributes to the community, sits on boards, improvisational cook. Seeks kind, hearty, worldly, competent man 45–57— mature yet young at heart.

Comparing the forthright, proud, accomplished person reflected in the second ad with the pitiful self-image and the totally unrealistic love object of my youthful longing, I am painfully reminded of how deeply the fairy-tale fantasy was ingrained when many of the women now looking for part- ners started out. Back then, we had such a weak self-image that we could only hope someone would "choose" us. Our dreams of love and romance were constructed out of received fantasies, not our own wants and needs. We chose partners who, we hoped, had the power to make our dream come true. We *needed* them to make life happen. As one woman put it, in contrast to her past expectations, her new understanding of love "feels deliberate and not desperate."

Eileen, a spirited entrepreneur, is now aware of how will- ingly she had given away her self in the early years of her marriage. Part of redefining intimacy—and recalibrating her marriage—was reclaiming her agency in the world. "Like many women of my generation, I stayed home to rear our children," she begins. "My husband was the sole breadwinner and used to frequently refer to the 'Golden Rule' of that time: 'He who makes the gold makes the rules!'" Then, she goes on, she dared to go out into the world, despite his displeasure. "I returned to school to get my master's degree. Although terrified, I realized I could do well. In fact, my first paper in nearly twenty years came back with a big red A+ and I received straight As all through school. This boosted my confidence in a major way."

The changes rippled out into the rest of her life. "Aside from making me feel better about myself, school was a fertile hotbed of interaction with other women my age. (It was a university geared to working adults.) And I entered what I now refer to as 'the age of rage,'" but there was no turning back. "I think women who were caregivers all their lives and deferred their own wants and needs can tend to go a bit overboard when they get back in touch with themselves." Once Eileen had done the hard work of making contact with herself, the party of the first part, it was almost easy to renegotiate the contract with her husband.

For Rosie too, the shift from neediness to self-reliance started with establishing an alliance with herself. "I used to think my love was defined by how much the other person cared for me. Honey, that is not the case. You can't receive real bona fide love until you love YOU." Now she sees intimacy from a new perspective. "I'm happy to say my new husband makes me hotter than a hot flash and our intimacy goes well beyond the bedroom. He is someone totally different. Why? Because thirty years ago I thought with my heart and not with my head. I saw what I wanted to see in my ex—and what I didn't like I thought I could change. You can't change anyone but yourself. I had to learn that lesson."

Another lesson women are learning (or relearning) is that there is no guarantee that love on our own terms will be any more carefree or long-lasting than love based on neediness. Many of the stories I heard ended in disappointment and pain, but even those mostly featured a woman who held her own. She came away battered but unbowed, marveling at the realization that she had loved in a way that was fresh and life-affirming.

Patricia, for one, met "the love of her life" online, and things became intense quickly. "He was so perfect," she recalls, "in the way he communicated, sexually and verbally and on the written page. Almost as important as the physical part was the fact that he could talk to me over the phone or write me a one-line e-mail and I would fall in love all over again." But the relationship faltered. For one thing, her daughter, who was fifteen, didn't like the idea of her mother dating, let alone forming a partnership. But after they were together for more than a year, a "partner" is what he claimed he wanted. In hindsight, his offer to sell his house and move in with her suggested to Patricia that part of the partnership would have been financial—"to pay off his ex-wife." As much as she thought she loved him, Patricia knew that something essential was missing; at a gut level she simply didn't trust him. Without that, any kind of long-lasting interdependence (financial or otherwise) was out of the question.

Over the two years they were together, however, Patricia blossomed. She got her body in shape, cut her dark blond hair into a stylish shoulder length, and bought more youthful—way *too* youthful, her kids complained—clothes. When it was over, Patricia was "heartbroken. In addition to falling madly in love at fifty, I also experienced the exquisite pain when it didn't work out." But she doesn't regret the relationship or the choices she made—for her children, against the "partnership"—based on her own good sense. As she put it to her daughter, who is now twenty-one, "I only hope you have as great a love as I had in your life. I wish that you have it with a husband, but I wouldn't have missed this time of my life for anything!"

OLD HABITS ARE HARD TO BREAK

Maryanne's story is a cliff-hanger. Each time I spoke to her she was more or less holding on to her fledgling sense of self. Soon after she and her husband of twenty-four years got divorced, she broke free. "I keep surprising myself," she says about being on her own, "with several decisions that seem almost as if another force outside my familiar self carries me to these new places of thinking, sensing, willing, and taking action. It is a very liberating process, though at times scary." She moved to a new city, enrolled in graduate school, and, she adds with a grin, "I got myself a Latin lover—an amazing salsa dancer, among many things, thirteen years younger, and a wonderful soul." And the sex: "It is so unlike me and my 'normal' tastes and inclinations. Antonio has an expertise in everything physical he does and very little inhibition (which I adore). . . . The fact that there is always an unexpected surprise sexually, his unanticipated sexual repertoire no matter how simple or elaborate is tapping into my sense of adventure and wonder. I appreciate that he's also very respectful of how I feel while he's choosing his . . . strategies."

At first, the boundaries were clear and acceptable to Mayanne. Antonio, who doesn't speak English very well, doesn't "ask any personal questions and he won't offer any personal information unless he's asked. He's someone who guards his independence and watches out for signals of emotional 'danger' or entanglement." Maryanne admired his gallantry. "His incredible quality of maintaining distances with unspoken, not-hurtful ways, is remarkable."

Soon, though, the narrative changed for Maryanne, and she found herself struggling not to fall back into romantic neediness and fantasy. "I'm now falling for this man. There is a strong connection between us (though he is totally unaware of this)." Sex for its own sake was morphing into an age-old scenario, for which the price has always been high. "I soon realized that he had more control over me. . . . I only see him when *he* wants. He declines my invitations for music performances that he would have loved. In other words, there is no room for dating. It's purely sexual and conversational between us. That's all." That was all she had signed on for, but her desire to enjoy is giving way to the desire to please—neediness. "I never ask for anything more and don't want him to think I am pressuring him. The more I like him, the harder it becomes to keep this thing just an affair, but when he comes to me, it's like the sun enters my home and my soul and I'm so grateful that the perfection of this amazingly beautiful body and his incredible sweetness shares my bed, my body, and my home. Then he leaves and I can hold on to the joy for about twenty-four hours before I start feeling unsettled and sad." Still, she adds, "I am trying very hard not to have more expectations and lose my sense of self into this turmoil."

Almost a year later, I heard from her again. "I'm seeing someone these days," Maryanne announced. He is a businessman and closer to her age. They were about to take a trip to Europe together. "It's fun," she concludes, "but I will never forget my wonderful young lover, who has opened the door for me and the way I view my sexuality." Although she feared that she would lose herself in that relationship, it set her free.

"He has helped me liberate my mind and body from old habitual behaviors and dead-end expectations."

Maryanne and Eileen and women like them are struggling within themselves to devise a mutually nurturing emotional vocabulary for the give-and-take of intimacy. In doing so, in daring to explore "the wilder shores of love," they are testing their own wants and needs and evolving a personal understanding of interdependence. They are also defying the public discomfort and the conventional wisdom that the prospects for romance—and sex—decline as a woman ages. On the contrary, women who are opening themselves to new ways of loving and finding new wells of feeling and experience are going for *more, not less.* Some want more intense sex while some are enjoying more intense companionship; others feel a need to establish boundaries for more solitude. Still others find that their relationships create opportunities for self-discovery (as well as, of course, self-doubt). Most report more focused commitment to a special few—and, yes, more loss. And most of those who are in long-term marriages report more turmoil—and, hopefully, growth. They are taking more risks and taking more control. And having more fun.

In each case, though, what makes it possible for a woman to want more and get more is a starting point of independence; from there on, whether or not to go for interdependence—and how much—depends on the circumstances. Debbie, who is fifty-six, has gone all the way, but her account sums up the New

Intimacy as well as anyone I talked to. "Women my age are old enough and experienced enough not to be blindsided, but young enough to feel the sweep of passion," she says. "Love at this stage allows me freedom—to be me, but also to recognize when I'm in the wrong. I trust my heart and my head that I am going in the right direction. The physical relationship," she adds, "has never been better—no fears of getting pregnant, kids walking in, et cetera. It's a wonderful place to be— no drama, lots of passion on all levels, an intellectual, emotional, and physical connection that really puts a smile on my face each day!"

It's too bad that *interdependence* is such a clunky word, because it so accurately describes the framework that supports the new love contracts we are entering into. Debbie's daily smile reflects a relationship built on give-and-take, respect, and trust. The New Intimacy is about creating the right amalgam of boundaries and vulnerability. It is about articulating needs, not answering neediness. It is about authenticity. It is about appreciation, not idolization. It is both measured and joyous. And it couldn't come at a better time.

Chapter 3

Undressing in the Dark

old body   old body in which somewhere
between crooked toe and forgetful head
the flesh encounters soul . . .

—Grace Paley, "One of the Softer Sorrows of Age"

I don't know a woman over fifty, though I would like to meet some, who would say she loves her body. Instead we love the bodies of airbrushed people we don't know or our own younger bodies—which we didn't love nearly so much back then. Like many of us, I look at pictures of myself at eighteen or thirty and think, What a pretty girl, only to remember that at the time I was totally disgusted by how "fat" I was. It is not surprising that after a lifetime of being brutally critical about our every cell and hair follicle, we aren't about to muster much acceptance for what is happening to our bodies now. The years of comfort inside our own skins we have lost are a waste that we can't reverse, but we can make peace with the (hopefully) strong, healthy bodies we have now; like aging, which we can't reverse either, we can engage with the process. As one woman commented upon seeing how good she looked in photographs taken ten years ago, "I realized that I'd better start appreciating how good I look now, because in ten more years I won't look this good either."

Now, I feel as "bad about my neck" as the next woman, and I certainly don't like the fact that the skin on my arms looks a whole lot more like the skin on my ninety-four-year-old mother's arms than my twenty-four-year-old daughter's. I am bemused every time I learn of another unexpected side effect of aging, like the information that because our lips get thinner and our brows get lower, we look mad even when we are feeling benign. And, god knows, I have enjoyed countless laughs at the expense of my accumulating bodily malfunctions. At the same time, I cherish the good feeling I have about my life these days, which has a lot to do with acceptance, freedom, and authenticity. Can I bring that equanimity to bear on my image in the mirror?

Although many of us are more fit and healthy than ever before in our lives, and many are reveling in the way our bodies are responding sexually, we can't seem to connect the flesh and blood that is functioning so effectively with the image we see in the mirror. What we see are the wrinkles and sags that horrified us back when we caught a glimpse of an older woman in a dressing room. It ain't a pretty picture. The best we can do is laugh. Meryl Streep captured that all-in-good-fun response in the movie *It's Complicated* when, the morning after a roll in the hay with her former husband, he waddles off in all his fleshy glory to the bathroom, and she rushes to cover herself. When he points out that they were both naked the night before, she replies, "Things look different lying down." Ha-ha.

But when the humor turns to self-contempt, it doesn't work for me. In an anthology of essays entitled *In the Fullness of Time: 32 Women on Life After 50,* one writer, Elizabeth Frank, talks about "the knowledge all aging women eventually have: that your vagina dries out unless you fill it with estrogen tablets and great goopy shots of Replens; that your pubic hair migrates from your balding pudendum to your face in the form of coarse black wires that require constant plucking if you are not to develop the mustache and eyebrows of a Civil War general," and so it goes. There is a lot of humor and countless birthday cards that embrace this tone, so I guess it works for some, but to me it is school-yard taunting and cruel. I can't help feeling that it is more an expression of self-loathing than of wit. Instead I am aiming for the same level of appreciation we often apply to other aspects of aging: This living, breathing body is better than the alternative.

Françoise Sagan, the iconoclastic French novelist of our youth, captured the conundrum we wrestle with. "There is a certain age when a woman must be beautiful to be loved, and then there comes a time when she must be loved to be beautiful." If we suspect that that is even a little true, how do we go about becoming loved for ourselves—and by ourselves?

Another essay in the same collection as Frank's—this one by Katherine Weissman, entitled "It Figures"—looks at her lifelong "war with my body" through a wider lens. "Encountering it in my sixties is like meeting an old enemy who has, unaccountably and regrettably, acquired new weapons since we last crossed paths." To outwit that Medusa, Weissman decides to look her in the eye. She signs up for a life drawing class and establishes a ritual of drawing herself naked every day. In class, she begins to appreciate the aesthetics of the older, fuller models: "they had substantial thighs; big squishy rear ends; generous breasts to which the word *perky* would never be applied. . . . They had weight and lusciousness and a certain courage and pride that more conventionally beautiful bodies did not." With quintessential woman-to-woman humor, she adds, "Of course, maybe I liked those models because they allowed me to feel superior."

In the course of her study of the female body Weissman achieves a profound insight. "I think human beings have difficulty seeing themselves as part of the natural world rather than above it. (That would imply, among other things, that we die)," she writes. "Drawing the body is a way to make the connections, to feel in our very bones that our physical selves are not for judging (no one would disparage a massive, elderly oak or an older lion that had, perhaps, put on a bit of weight now that he had retired from hunting) but for perceiving." What, exactly, is there to perceive about our aging bodies?

GETTING UNDER OUR OWN SKIN

The female body at fifty or sixty is a natural wonder that can perform feats of daring and strength. My friend Joanne is a continuing inspiration. Back when she was forty, she was a workaholic who rarely saw the light of day, let alone the fluorescent light of a gym; she was so into her head that I doubt she would have recognized her own body if it was walking toward her. But when she was sixty-five, she completed her first (age-appropriate) triathlon. In between, she spent vacations on rugged Earthwatch expeditions—in Namibia, in Kenya, and in the peat bogs of Ireland; she started her own business documenting the stories of real people for the not-for-profits who serve them; and she has sustained a wide circle of friends whom she has nurtured and who have been at her side through good times and bad.

The transformative factor has been the discovery of a joyful "fitness and lifestyle" program called the Nia Technique when she was fifty. Regular workouts, which she describes as "a cardiovascular blend of dance and martial arts (that is also a lot of fun)" have given her her body back—or, in her case, ownership for the first time. "Nia is a permanent part of my life," she says, "for three big reasons—my body, my spirit, and my mind . . . pretty much in that order." She can now "bound down the stairs, which used to hurt my knees, and," she says, "I can touch my toes." At the same time, she is respectful of the wear and tear on her body. "When I get out of bed in the morning, I am not so nimble," she admits. So she has established a regimen that keeps her flexible and fit. "When I am eighty-five I want to bike and swim and do another triathlon."

I have no intention of training for a triathlon of any kind, but I could imagine someone like me attempting at least some of the course (the bike ride, maybe) she completed. A far cry from the Iron Man model, it recognizes the limitations of an aging body while celebrating the amazing things it can still accomplish. Organized by a sixty-two-year-old triathlon legend named Sally Edwards, the course is a .25-mile swim, a 9-mile bike ride, and a 3.1-mile run. Joanne trained twice a week with twenty others, one of whom was a "large" woman who didn't have a bike, hadn't run for years due to painful knees, but was determined to get into shape. She completed the race alongside Joanne. "What does it mean to feel good about your body?" Joanne mused. "To me it means feeling strong and healthy and optimistic, knowing I can meet the challenges I set for myself."

Dr. James Fries, who studies aging athletes, has a glass-half-full take on late bloomers like Joanne. Most athletes peak at an early age and spend the rest of their lives trying to ward off physical decline, he points out, while someone who starts training at sixty can take advantage of the "plasticity of aging" and become faster as she ages; at seventy she won't run like a twenty-five-year-old, but she will have made progress since she was sixty.

Feeling strong and healthy and optimistic is also an aphrodisiac. However they look, our bodies are capable of great sex till the day we die. What stands in the way of exploring that delicious prospect with abandon is the cultural distaste for the image of sex among "seniors" that undermines our appreciation of our bodies and what they are capable of. Nevertheless, older women are breaking free of social restrictions and their own past limitations. The pull of gravity notwithstanding, our bodies are performing sexually in wondrous ways; despite the dearth of partners, the connections women are making are various and inventive. Despite shriveled orifices and waning hormones, the old girl has never had more juice.

TURNING ON TO OUR SEXUALITY

Nowhere is the dividing line between half empty and half full more complex physiologically and more shrouded in mythology and confusion than in our sexuality. As Frank's essay proclaims, we all have a pretty good understanding of the physiological changes that affect our sex lives, and it is easy to attribute a range of afflictions to aging. A study of more than thirty-one thousand women between the ages of forty-five and sixty-four found that 44 percent of them reported a problem with desire, arousal, or orgasm. Many of those women have resigned themselves to disappointment, even though their problems may be caused by many things that have nothing to do with age—from interactions among the accumulating medications we are taking to chronic yeast infections to thyroid and testosterone deficiency to various health- and psychology-related conditions. Many of them are treatable, and others can be circumvented.

In view of the fact that desire in women is stoked by myriad psychological, emotional, and physical triggers (including simply being desired), a reduction of heat from one source still leaves many others. Martha Meana, a professor of psychology, likens the difference between male and female desire to two control panels, one with a single on/off switch, the other with numerous knobs and dials.

The decline of estrogen is the universal factor affecting midlife sexuality, but the symptoms vary with each woman; most of them can be dealt with. Estrogen replacement therapy is still controversial, but many women are committed to it. The vaginal dryness caused by hormone depletion can be treated too, as Frank's essay points out so graphically. The other causes of painful intercourse include changes in the vaginal wall and the clitoris. Many women find that experimenting with positions and stimulation not only solves the pain problem but creates exciting new sources of pleasure. The sex act itself can contribute to the well-being that fosters good sex. An orgasm releases hormones, such as endorphins, that stimulate the immune system—and enhance sleep (later)—and a surge of oxytocin, which is a great pain and stress reliever. Overall, the cardiovascular workout itself is as beneficial as a set of tennis.

Unlike tennis, though, a partner is not required in order to be sexually fit. Women without opportunities for regular sex and those who simply enjoy pleasuring themselves consider masturbation a delightful option, yet only half as many women over fifty as men report masturbating regularly, according to a study published in the *New England Journal of Medicine*. To enhance the experience, many doctors—especially women doctors—urge a regular vaginal workout. Kegel exercises, the tightening (as if you are trying to stop urinating) and releasing of the pubococcygeus muscle—located at the base of the pelvic floor—are recommended highly by sex therapists and spiritualists alike. Gina Ogden, who is both, is a big fan. "Kegels increase the muscle tone in your vagina and strengthen your pelvic floor muscles, which support your bladder, uterus, and rectum," she explains. (And, we should note, may forestall peeing when you sneeze.) "All this toning has the potential to make your physical orgasms deeper, stronger, and more satisfying," says Ogden. Moreover, she believes, the exercise is "a consciousness-raising activity." Regular practice "can act like a kind of 'vagina monologue' to increase your relationship with the part of you that's usually kept under wraps, hidden and silent."

Many women arrive at Second Adulthood with their sexuality still, or again, "hidden and silent." And they come sexually alive only after they get there. But more and more of us are getting there. Based on the hundreds of interviews she did for *Sex and the Seasoned Woman,* Gail Sheehy reports that "a great many women are finding 'middlesex' more enjoyable than married life ever was in their thirties and forties when juggling jobs, motherhood, and what's-for-dinner guilt made for mostly exhausted sex." Many are finding a deepening intimacy even as time has its way with their bodies. Married to her second husband for seventeen years, Margo has seen the relationship blossom "into mature love and intimacy. He is my best friend. At nearly fifty-nine years old, I have discovered that these are the best days of my life, in every way. Sure, I would like to have a little nip and tuck here and there, but I feel good in my skin, and my husband has no trouble touching it, regardless of how much skin there is. Now, if we only had more time to make love."

THE LANGUAGE OF LOVE

What Margo calls "mature love and intimacy," Dr. Robert Butler, author of *The New Love and Sex After 60,* calls a "second language" of sex, "which is emotional and communicative as well as physical." It is "learned rather than instinctive and is often vastly underdeveloped since it depends upon the ability to recognize and share feelings in words, actions, and unspoken perception, and to achieve mutual tenderness and thoughtfulness with another person." It takes a long-term commitment to become fluent, he adds. "It is a slow-developing aptitude, acquired deliberately and painstakingly through years of experience in giving and receiving."

As we keep discovering, our bodies speak through the thinking mind and the feeling mind at the same time. The "language" that Butler describes parallels the communication system that scientists are calling "limbic resonance"—"a symphony of mutual exchanges and internal adaptation whereby two mammals become attuned to each other's inner states." Rising from the most primitive part of the brain, limbic resonance synchronizes the menstrual cycles of roommates and enables lovers to modulate each other's hormonal status, immune function, and even sleep patterns. We can literally miss a loved one so much that it hurts.

The authors of *A General Theory of Love,* where limbic resonance is explained, go on to show how good vibes make for interdependence between lovers. We often see love as "the art of the deal," they argue, in which one good deed deserves another; but the "physiology of love" is a reciprocity "wherein each person meets the needs of the other, because neither can provide for his own. Such a relationship is not 50-50—it's 100-100."

Sandi didn't find that limbic resonance in her first marriage, but when she fell in love again all systems clicked in. "I never knew love and sex could be so wonderful, and this after my ex had termed me 'frigid' over the last several years of marriage!" she enthuses. "Sometimes we make love all night or for a few hours in the morning. We spend half the week together and half apart, which certainly keeps the passion and chemistry sparking." The only turnoff is the real estate bust. "We are married in our hearts and minds and will take that real step when the real estate market turns around and we can sell our separate houses to buy one together."

There are many women for whom better sex is not more sex or even sex with penetration. One, who has been married close to forty years, told me that while she and her husband "pleasure each other" only about once a month, her orgasms (and his too) are bigger and longer than at any point in their marriage—including their honeymoon. Sometime, she admits, she wonders what it would be like with a new partner. "It might be more exciting," she says, "but it couldn't be more satisfying."

GETTING WHAT WE WANT

Another reason the generation of women who lived through the "sexual revolution" may be getting better sex now is that for many, the wild sixties weren't all that much fun—social pressure, inexperience, and mixed moral messages often inhibited their enjoyment, if not their sexual activity. But, most of all, sex gets better as a woman begins to acknowledge what she wants—even if what she wants is to explore the unknown—and feels entitled to get it. After a lifetime of dedication to pleasing others in every respect, including sex—and including faking it—the autonomy and authority we are accumulating in Second Adulthood gives us the wherewithal to ask ourselves, "Am *I* enjoying this?" and, if not, to do something about it.

"For the first time in the last thirty-four years I am actually savoring, enjoying, participating, reaching climaxes every time," Theresa wrote me. What makes the difference? "This time my enjoyment comes first. I feel young, energized, the serotonin levels are high, and it's such a wonderful feeling." She is in a relationship where "age-wise (he is more than twenty-five years younger), financially, socially, nothing matches. This time around there are no expectations, no binding, no 'Let's get married'! Been there, done that! I savor my freedom and will not be bogged down. Are we compatible? Can I meet his desires? Is the sex comfortable for me

considering our ages and the biological changes in me? YES!"
Her passion and freedom are a turn-on to both of them.

Many women still carry a lot of baggage, and it still gets in
the way. Throughout her twenties Winnie had lots of sex and
lots of guilt. "My body loved the sensations, but my mind said
it was bad." She married at twenty-six "for all the wrong reasons" and "hated having sex with my husband. This time I felt
guilty because I was NOT having sex." After twenty years she
divorced him and "met the perfect man for me, and the sex was
out of this world. We were both love- and sex-starved, and this
combination must have been a catalyst for our sexual enjoyment. For the first time in my life I truly ENJOYED SEX!!!"

Ironically, just when things were getting good for her, her
partner gave out. "I think it is low libido and erectile dysfunction on his part," she speculated in a post on the VibrantNation Web site. The more expressive and experimental women
become, the more they find themselves having to deal, like
Winnie, with their same-aged partners' problems. Men experience hormonal and physical changes, but because for them
performance depends on a well-functioning penis (the "on/
off switch"), the prospect of such obvious "failure" can turn
a man off. In the absence of a circle of trust to confide in, he
may just give up, even though the condition may be completely treatable.

In the same way that estrogen depletion can make it
harder for women to become aroused, a falloff of testoster-

one production can reduce desire in men (a small dose of testosterone can do the trick for both men and women). Vascular changes can reduce the capacity of the penis to become engorged with blood, and an enlarged prostate can inhibit ejaculation, which is why it takes many older men longer to climax than it used to. Health conditions, medications, and depression (the suicide rate for men over sixty is high in relation to the general population and getting higher at an alarming rate) can all undercut a man's interest in sex. So can emotional turmoil in the relationship. Frank talk among women on this taboo subject—the kind of talk our generation has perfected—is contributing to a first step toward treatment: frank talk between partners.

Winnie's post elicited some voices of experience, who shared their advice and reassurance. Laura had also been surprised, she wrote, when she and her husband "deeply in love; best friends (with a sense of humor) in sync with life, including sex, hit a brick wall! The truth—we believed we were invincible. First we had to stop being angry at our own issues with getting older, which made us not very nice to each other." They got through it, and, she adds, "I am pretty sure the ace in the hole was our sense of humor!"

Alice's lover had erectile dysfunction too, she wrote, but truth telling on his part enabled them to explore new frontiers of intimacy. He is "quite honest about that issue, making it a nonissue; as he says, 'the equipment doesn't always work, but I still love to pleasure you.'" And he does. "He has gifted me with the understanding that lovemaking at this stage (sixty-five and sixty-four) is really 'pleasuring' each other and that there are many ways (manual, oral, vaginal) to have full-blown satisfaction over the hours we spend in the throes of passion."

"I finally got the courage to really talk to him about his ED," Winnie reported back to her online advisers, "and he finally got the courage to share his fears and embarrassment with me. We decided to keep trying together to bring back the romance, and he agreed to see a doctor in the future if necessary." Three weeks after that conversation, "even though we've both been suffering from colds and sinus infections . . . we're closer than ever and look forward to our next 'rendezvous.' By the way, a bubble bath, candlelight, soft music, and massages work wonders for the libido!"

When a superstud like Michael Douglas, sixty-five, touts the benefits of Viagra, you know that the stigma attached to discussing ED is waning. Indeed, the arrival of the drug has revived the sex life for many couples; and it has enabled many single men—including "condo Romeos," so called because of the carrying-on in retirement communities—to have lively sex lives. But a lot of women are underwhelmed. One was bowled over when her husband, with whom she had not had sex for years, came home from the pharmacy a newly minted satyr. She found his advances an abuse of power, especially because she hadn't been consulted before he made his decision. Ultimately his insensitivity disrupted the delicate balance of acceptance in their marriage and led to divorce. Another told me she just feels "used" because her husband seems to be turned on by the medication rather than her. Without the ingredients of mutuality and trust, even the most powerful elixirs will undermine, not enhance, sexual interdependence. And if those ingredients are present, the sex act is less important for intimacy than tenderness and respect are.

SEX, LOVE, AND LUST

Love, lust, sex, and intimacy involve many states of mind and body, and they can combine in countless ways that in their variety reflect the New Intimacy—sometimes even in one blissful relationship. But when they don't, some women I have talked to are choosing to mix and match rather than lose out. A groundbreaking study of women's extramarital affairs, *The Erotic Silence of the American Wife,* by Dalma Heyn, profiled numerous women who broke the adultery taboo without destroying their marriages. Since 1992, when her book came out, further studies report that women are catching up to men in the infidelity department—though we are still way behind. To which science writer Natalie Angier, reporting on the phenomenon, had this to say: "The fidelity gap may be explained more by cultural pressures than any real differences in the sex drives of men and women. Men with multiple partners typically are viewed as virile, while women are considered promiscuous."

The response to Heyn's book confirms Angier's insight. It was barely reviewed and was dismissed even by "professionals," because, in the opinion of psychologist Carol Gilligan, its findings were too hot to handle. CC's story is typical. She is married to Martin and having an affair with Stephen. Sex with Martin had always been unsatisfying. "My assumption," CC told Heyn, "was that this was the price for being loved and cared for." Then Second Adulthood brought CC the hot flash that she was entitled to call her share of the shots. "What I didn't understand at the time was how much the word 'sex' was limited to what he wanted and precluded what I wanted." Sex with Stephen, when he entered the picture, was just what she wanted. Did that spell the end of her marriage? "No, just the opposite," she says. "My marriage feels better to me now than it has in ten years. My marriage might *stay* because I'm getting good sex!" She loves Martin and she believes that he loves her, but the place of her marriage—and the men—in her life has shifted. "I've come to see that what's most important is not just to make the *marriage* work, but to make my life—which includes my marriage—work for me. . . . My marriage can't be my priority; *I* have to be. And now I am. And it works for me."

Why is this situation so threatening to so many? Probably because, as Heyn concludes, women's extramarital relationships represent a departure "from idealized models of femininity and masculinity, and to the return of easy, comfortable, unidealized relationships." Why is it so appealing to the Second Adulthood women who are doing it? For the same reasons.

Heyn identifies a second, intriguing dynamic among her subjects—an "odd correlation between getting chronologically older while simultaneously losing a feeling of being a 'grown-up.'" This "sexual anomaly" occurs when "after many years of marriage, women feel 'old' but not 'adult'—while in their affairs, they felt 'adult' but not 'old.'"

"Monogamy is my way," says Lolly, regardless of sexual activity. Now seventeen years into her third marriage—the first lasted sixteen years ("he was a devoted dad, but not a devoted husband"); the second, under a year—"The meaning of love has changed for me," she says. Reading M. Scott Peck's *The Road Less Traveled* clarified her thinking. "He says 'love is a decision,' not a feeling. That helped me get off the roller-coaster ride of needing to feel 'in love.'" Her current husband, she says, "has been wonderful for me in midlife, supportive of my desire for education and personal growth. He represents stability, which is what I needed." The problem is that the "passion that I once felt for my husband has gone away. We have a sexless relationship."

Which is not to say that her sexuality is being neglected. Physically she takes care of herself. "My sex life is solo," she says. Chemically, she is reassured, all systems are go. "I am amazed when I occasionally meet a guy who turns on the juice in me. Wow! It's great to know it's still there." But the most lively component of her sexuality is her imagination. "I've wondered about experiencing sex with a woman. If I survive my husband, perhaps that's an option. I've fantasized about an affair, but even just the fantasy interferes with my busy life. It isn't worth it. My mother had a love affair that began in her seventies with a man twenty years younger (which freaked out my husband, who was only a couple of years younger than him). But that puts a spark in my eye for my later years."

While Lolly is able to enjoy her sexuality without marital sex, Kate can't even reach her sexuality anymore. Any pleasure she ever took in her body has been banished by a sexual crisis in her marriage that turned on every woman's worst nightmare—how her looks had changed. When she and her husband of thirty years began having trouble in bed, they tried the usual solutions, including Viagra, but none worked for long. "Then one day he told me that *I* was the problem," she says. "He told me that he no longer found me sexually attractive. That I had gained weight and it turned him off. . . . The most humiliating of all is when he told me that if he watched me performing oral sex on him, it made his penis go soft." She was stunned, even more so when he tried to sell her on the idea that his cruelty was for her own good.

"He thought by telling me these things I would lose weight. He thought he was doing me a favor by telling me these things." Four years later, they "talk and laugh a lot," but she hasn't been "in the mood" since, despite counseling and her husband's repeated apologies and protestations of love. "Now who am I punishing? Him? Myself? Will I continue to live this way?" Kate wonders. "I envy women who are involved with men who understand that bodies change and age over the years. Who love unconditionally."

LOVING AN AGING BODY

Photographer Sally Mann has been photographing bodies of all ages for years (she was criticized back in 1988 for using adolescent girls, and four years later, for using her own children, as models). Recently she undertook a daring exploration of unconditional love in the context of bodies that have changed. In her case it was her husband's body that was deteriorating; but the trust and mutual appreciation they showed each other is a profound expression of what it means to love—and be loved—body and soul. Over a period of six years she created an extraordinary collection of photographs of her husband's aging and, later, disease-ridden body. In an essay about the collection, she traces the relationship: "I have looked hard at my husband since the first long strides he took into the room where I was languishing on a ratty chenille couch in some student apartment. That was forty years

ago, and almost the first thing I did was photograph him."
The prospect of scrutinizing and photographing his decline
was, they both realized, fraught with painful possibilities of
exploitation, betrayal, shame. Yet they felt the project also
offered the possibility of a new level of intimacy in their long
relationship. "Before me lay a man as naked and vulnerable
as any wretch strung across the mythical vulture-topped
rock. At our ages, we are past the prime of life, given to sinew
and sag, and Larry bears, with his trademark godlike nobil-
ity, the further affliction of a late-onset muscular dystrophy.
That he was so willing is both heartbreaking and terrifying
at once." They worked together in her studio. "No phone, no
kids, two fingers of bourbon, the smell of the ether, the two
of us—still in love, still at work."

Her words go further than any I have read to evoke the
alchemy—the interdependence—that binds two aging bodies.

If midlife were an out-of-body experience or love were
blind, we might be able to get away without looking in the
mirror. But as things stand, we need to see ourselves straight
on through the lenses of health and strength, gratitude and
self-acceptance. As Charlotte put it at her seventy-fifth birthday party, "We are weather-beaten, but not browbeaten."

If any woman would find it hard to achieve that sense of
comfort in her own skin as it gives in to the years, it should
be a fifty-three-year-old fashion model. Joy Bell, one of the
few "mature" models who still gets jobs, has embraced her

no-longer-ingenue body, and consciously uses it to express a new confidence in being herself and looking her age. "There used to be a lot of jumping around," she says. "When I was young, they wanted a more passive, more malleable look." Now she strikes "a confident pose, two feet firmly on the ground. It's in the shoulders, the way you stand. It's a 'you know who you are' look." That is a body language we can all speak.

It is hard to learn to appreciate your body as it stands there in your mirror—the comparisons to ads for clothes and cosmetics and the youthful icons around us are painful. (I confess that I see the day approaching when I won't want to appear in a bathing suit.) But the bigger picture tells another story; inside that body you are walking, dancing, having good sex, and exuding good health. That sounds pretty attractive to me. Many of the women I quote in this chapter— more than average in the general population, I'm sure—have been able to rebuild their self-image by gaining confidence about the whole shape of their lives; for them, the good feeling about being the age they are has engendered goodwill toward, if not the aesthetics of their body, its capacity for accomplishment and joy.

Chapter 4

Cyberspace—Where the Action Is

We are, all of us, calling and calling across the incalculable
gulfs which separate us . . .

—David Grayson, *Adventures in Friendship*

The Internet has had an impact on just about every kind of
intimacy we are nourishing in our Second Adulthood. In
fact, it is safe to say that the tools and experiences of connecting online make many of the dynamic and inventive
relationships we are enjoying possible. Instead of having to
call twenty former classmates for an address (perhaps outdated) of another, we Google that person (no one even has to
know that we are curious to reconnect); sure, it has always
been possible to find people and information we are looking

for, but now we can do it on a whim. Instead of sitting home waiting—for an invitation, for a call from a doctor who may or may not take the time to tell us about what we have, for the sound of a human voice—we sit at our computers in communion with the world.

We are online at all hours, expressing the widest range imaginable of needs and feelings, from seeking out old lovers to Skyping with grandchildren to raising issues too sensitive even for friends about sexuality, parenting, and "bad thoughts" to coordinating parent care with siblings to reaching out for human contact to ordering the supplies that make it possible to sustain a homebound life. Our age group came late to the new technology, but now we are among the most active Internet users. According to recent data, women over forty-five are the group showing the greatest growth in social networking. Over-fifty users—men and women— doubled in 2009. (While nearly half of men visit sex-themed sites, more than one-third of women of all ages do as well.) As a survey conducted by VibrantNation, an information-sharing Web site for women over fifty, points out, "Before the workplace revolution and the Internet, women's external connections declined as they aged. . . . As recently as a decade ago, women expected that as they crossed the threshold of 50+, they would become progressively marginalized from mainstream society." With one click we can venture out into an even larger world than we knew before we crossed that threshold birthday.

The Internet opens up a parallel universe where our existing relationships expand or take new turns, where we can become intimate with people we never see and explore experiences we never imagined would be available to us. It also, of course, creates new opportunities for betrayal and dishonesty and real danger. But for the most part, we revel in the openness of the conversations and the options for self-expression; we take risks by putting ourselves out there, and we protect ourselves by retaining veto power over overtures from out there. We can try on new personalities, put our beliefs to the test, and get that much closer to confirming our true selves.

Even with intimates, people we could just as easily meet for coffee or call on the phone, we can communicate online with more thought, fewer distractions, and in wider circles at once. At this stage of life for this generation, the nature of any community we are part of is very much dependent on being linked in. And as the gerontologists keep reminding us, an active social network is a key to healthy aging. The Internet supports both the independence and the interdependence that are vital to the way we love now.

Whenever we break ranks with traditional expectations for women our age, as we are doing now by exploring the frontiers of intimacy, two big doubts hold us back: Am I the only one?

Am I crazy? An active Internet life soothes both. We need not be lonely, no matter how alone we are, and we need not stifle our "crazy" impulses; we can check them out with others who are always out there waiting to hear from us. We can even siphon off behaviors that might jeopardize cherished relationships. Author Carolyn Heilbrun, known for her crotchety behavior and impatience, delighted in letting off steam online. "If one sometimes feels compelled, as we all do, to complain about any dimension or all dimensions of one's life but does not do so because all the people one sees are sick of it and will visit even less often if complaints or criticism are forced upon them," she writes in *The Last Gift of Time: Life Beyond Sixty,* "well, there are people out there who will be happy to exchange complaints and perhaps even help to talk us out of them, or counter them with other, strange grievances."

INTIMACY WITHOUT PROXIMITY

My friend Amanda, who has always maintained a wide circle of friends, now carries out several close relationships—long-standing ones as well as brand-new ones—in cyberspace. She became computer-literate for her job running a small organization, but it was only about eight years ago that she began to use it "as a personal tool." When she retired from full-time work, the hours she spent online carried her across the chasm separating her dear colleagues left behind in the office from her new home-based consulting business.

She revived old friendships and even made an important new friend, the mother of a woman she knew. They had met occasionally at the daughter's home and enjoyed chatting. "She is twenty years older than I am, but she is so funny—she has a wicked sense of humor—such a good listener, and has such an interesting story," Amanda says. They bonded by e-mail. "It all began when my son was having his meltdown," she explains. "I was having lunch with my friend, and when I told her what was happening she said, 'I probably shouldn't be telling you this, but my mother is going through the same thing with my brother.' He had been a heroin user, was clean for seven years, and had just gone back on drugs. I asked if she thought I could write to her mother, she said yes, so I e-mailed her, saying, 'I gather we are both having the same heartbreak.'" A channel of profound intimacy was opened, almost without the usual getting-to-know-you phase, between people who rarely see each other or talk on the phone.

"She wrote back full of insight and self-knowledge and all the things you think about when a kid is in trouble," Amanda recalls. Now they talk almost daily, about their lives, their interests, their feelings. Amanda looks forward to what her new friend has to say; she has nearly given up journaling, because the e-mail conversation is similarly open and full of self-discovery. "Every time we had a childhood memory we would share it. Once she wrote me, 'I can't believe we are shar-ing all the emotional slugs we are finding by turning over these emotional rocks. I wonder why we're doing this. Does it mean anything?' 'We are doing it because we can,'" Amanda says she replied. "You can talk about things in e-mail that you can't over lunch," she tells me, "and you can go on as long as you want—even a shrink cuts you off at fifty minutes. E-mail erases time, but it also expands time. Each of us has the time to talk, free-associate, without watching the other person's eyes glaze over, in ways we never could under normal circumstances." There is another option for self-discovery in their correspondence that Amanda's online friend identified. "I can't believe I have written you all this. You probably won't even get to the end," she wrote. "But it will help me when I reread it."

Amanda's e-mail network includes a friend who lives in England—"It erases distance and time zones"—and another who is a night owl—"She is up till four A.M, I go to sleep at nine o'clock; there is almost no time we could talk on the phone." Her sister, whose "muttering and ditzy diction" drove Amanda crazy in person, is much easier to relate to in e-mails. And even if something her sister does drives Amanda crazy, her sister can't see the faces she is making. They have become closer than they have ever been. Amanda has also found the courage to confront toxic relationships with a well-crafted e-mail. She has one piece of advice for those who get real online. "Write what you want to say, but don't put the address on until you are sure you want to send it." We all fear hitting an unintentional SEND.

Is Amanda's disembodied circle of trust different from the old-fashioned kind? Psychiatrist Michael Civin calls these "Internet-mediated relationships." In his book *Male Female e-mail: The Struggle for Relatedness in a Paranoid Society*, he poses some challenging questions about what we gain and lose. "From the nearly infinite inside to the nearly infinite outside, we can reach out, we can be in touch. But to what are we reaching, and what is doing the reaching? What does it mean to be in touch when neither side can touch? And why have so many come to favor these infinite but disembodied alternatives to the palpable substance of human interactions?" Our online interactions call upon new communication skills at the same time as they disqualify some that we have relied upon.

LEARNING NEW WAYS TO "READ" ANOTHER PERSON

Civin's questions are particularly pertinent for women, who from early childhood are driven by a desire for, as Carol Gilligan puts it, "relationship or mutual understanding." Indeed, Gilligan, who has studied the cultural forces that shape women, finds a pattern of mixed messages that have confused us. "Girls are caught between their ability to read other minds and a culture that tells us we can't read other minds, between their empathy and desire for connection and a society that places a premium on separateness and independence." As we continue to work on resolving those conflicts well into Second Adulthood, we now have to also take into account how they play in cyberspace.

For example, our capacity for intimacy is enhanced by a sensitivity to the body language, or simply the "vibe," we get in the presence of another person. Picking up psychic cues is not possible when reading a computer screen. How does that affect the intimacy achieved? A study from the University of Michigan found that, measured by standard personality tests, today's college students score 40 percent lower than their counterparts twenty or thirty years ago on a questionnaire that assesses empathy. "The biggest drop," Ruth Marcus reports in the *Washington Post,* "occurred after the year 2000, coinciding with the rise of online communications and social networking." One author of the study, Sara Konrath, told *USA Today,* "Empathy is best activated when you can see another person's signal for help."

A similar if surprising point about empathy turns up in research done to assess the dangers of talking on even a hands-free phone while driving. Conversing with a disembodied voice is, the study concluded, a distraction that slows down the driver's reaction time. If, on the other hand, the person is in the adjoining seat, what goes on between them can enhance reaction time. For one thing, the passenger is watching the road almost as intently as the driver and can spot an imminent danger, even ahead of the driver. But here is the empathy part: When the road is dark or dangerous, both individuals instinctively mute their conversation, enabling—encouraging—the driver to concentrate and supplying wordless moral support. A friend talking from a different time zone and climate has no such function.

How does being physically present or absent affect the brain chemistry that fires women's finely tuned sensitivity to others? Many studies have shown that when we are together—working on a project, laughing over lunch—the intimacy drug oxytocin is released. By the same token, negative vibes—even a fleeting facial expression—can send a women reeling. "The female brain has a far more negative alert reaction to relationship conflict and rejection than does the male brain," writes Dr. Louann Brizendine in *The Female Brain*. "Conflict is more likely to set in motion a cascade of negative reactions, creating feelings of stress, upset and fear." When that happens the oxytocin level drops and the stress hormone cortisol takes over. The oxytocin spigot does not respond to faceless words on a screen in the same way.

Each of us has her own way of using this new tool. I, for one, hate talking on the phone; I don't much like long chatty e-mails either, but I love the efficiency of information exchange and the opportunity for a quick base touching. For staying in touch I prefer lunch. But this book wouldn't be as full of first-person anecdotes and totally honest insights if it weren't for the generosity of strangers who shared their lives with me online. Furthermore, while I was deprived of information about what they looked like and how they spoke, I got answers to questions I probably wouldn't have even dared ask in a classic face-to-face interview.

Computer relating has also enriched my relationship with my daughter under circumstances in which we might have grown apart. For the last six years she has lived far away, first in college and then in South America. In the first few years, we e-mailed, we instant-messaged, occasionally we talked on the phone. I quickly understood that each electronic form had its own level of intimacy; she expressed herself with varying degrees of accessibility depending on which technology she chose. E-mails were for information or to broach difficult subjects, like money. IMs were for more immediate and confidential exchanges. A phone call meant high drama was involved. Knowing the technological code enhanced my ability to read between the lines of our conversations. By the time she moved farther away, we were also able to video-chat regularly, which gave me the visual information I had been deprived of. Did she look pale or tired? Was her new haircut becoming? And wasn't her kitten adorable? When people asked me if I missed her, I had to acknowledge that I did, but I didn't feel that we were missing out on each other's lives.

A CIRCLE OF TRUST IN CYBERSPACE

For women like Amanda, who wants to choose her words and discount annoying habits, e-mail is much more satisfying than a phone call, but less satisfying than being together. For two other friends, the means of reaching out to a large circle of trust at a uniform level of intimacy and with more detail than would have been possible individually has given each of them a degree of support and consolation unimaginable in years past.

When her mother was in the final stages of her life, Ruthie left her Colorado home to be with her. To keep connected with her caring community, she sent an almost daily update to fifty family members and friends. They were long and writerly accounts, almost like old-fashioned letters. She reported medical developments of the day, and she shared the range of emotions that she was experiencing. It didn't feel like an impersonal mass mailing to those of us on the list; in fact, I was honored to be among her intimates. One e-mail, written when she was cleaning out the house her mother had lived in for fifty years, ended this way:

> So I now will hope to sleep. Bid you good night. Send you my love and thank you so much for yours. Your care and lovingness helps me remember I'm not alone though I am and must continue this journey and try to learn as much as I can. One day at a time. One hour at a time. One drawer at a time. One closet at a time.
>
> I love you each and all.

The wave of "lovingness" that she received from "each and all" sustained her throughout the ordeal. And the information she shared enabled us to be there for her in ways a hurried phone call could never have.

"As almost all of you know, Jenny suffered a stroke on Sunday," wrote Jane about her daughter. I didn't know. I felt terrible that I hadn't heard. So I was immensely grateful to receive the long and detailed account that Jane, a wonderful writer, sent out to her list. As I read the description of Jenny's status I found the typos to be poignant testimony—an online "signal for help"?—to what Jane was going through.

She continues to show amazing improvement every day, surprising her therapists and gladdening all our hearts. It is a very intensive program and she will be there for 2 more weeks, after which she'll be released to come home and continue pysical and speech therapy on an in-home and outpatient basis. The chances odf her making a full recovery grow brighter every day—in just a week in rehab she's progressed to be able to walk, albeit with a cane, transfer herself from bed to wheelchair to john without asistance, etc. She's left handed and the stroke primarily affected her right side, but she's regained the use of her hight leg and the right shoulder and arm—the hand is weak but getting stronger every day.

The next e-mail made it clear that the outpouring of support and concern the previous mailing generated had heartened both mother and daughter:

> To all of you who've called, emailed or otherwise contacted me—good news! Jenny came home from rehab today, 3 weeks after her stroke, and she is well on her way to making a full recovery! She can walk and talk, although she says she's not adding chewing gum to the list any time soon, and her sense of humor and optimism is intact. . . .
>
> I can't believe it's been only 3 weeks since it happened— it feels like three years, every day of which lasted a hundred hours! But I'm exhaling now, knowing that Jenny has a lot going for her—youth, strength, motivation and stubbornness, as well as a wonderful partner who's wholeheartedly devoted to supervising her recovery and a great and supportive group of friends. She's also had, and continues to have, the love and prayers of many, many people. Thank you for thinking of her, and of me, too.

Ruthie and Jane each brought her existing support group together online and deepened the intimacy between herself and each member of that group; many men and women are building entirely new communities the same way. Such virtual communities can forestall a serious pitfall of aging.

"One of the greatest challenges or losses that we face as older adults is not about our health, but it's actually about our social network deteriorating on us," says Joseph F Coughlin, director of the AgeLab at MIT. "The new future of old age is about staying in society, staying in the workplace, and staying very connected." The Internet "provides a way to make new connections, new friends and new senses of purpose."

THE KINDNESS OF STRANGERS

The collective support of strangers in the same boat has been of enormous help to women confronting the afflictions that strike our age group. Surveys have shown that women trust online medical advice more than they do the hurried or imperious recommendations from their doctors. In addition to moral support and crucial information, there are recovery benefits from belonging to such a community. A study from Ohio State University's Cancer Center found that breast cancer patients who participated in support groups increased their chances for survival. After seven years, the support group patients were 56 percent less likely to die than those who had been on their own. They also exhibited stronger immune systems, fewer side effects from the treatment, and less stress.

Less serious but no less supportive are some online offerings that bring women together to go somewhere or do something in real time that they would never do on their own. I'm no fan of the word *cougar* to describe midlife women on the make; it casts confident and assertive women as predatory and slightly ridiculous (and recalls that other undignified animal designation of our youth, the Playboy bunny). But it does offer a key word for women who don't mind the image and are curious about the experience.

Like the countless Web sites that speak to a particular group, Vacations for Cougars invites women over forty to travel to San Juan del Sur on the coast of Nicaragua for a week of sun, fun, and surf—and men. "It's a vacation hot spot in Nicaragua for surfers," the Web site explains. "So not only do you have all the men who live here, you also have a lot of tourists. My favorite saying," adds the founder, who chaperones the trips, "is 'not all crack is bad' because the surfers often wear their board shorts about an inch too low. Hard-bodied surfer crack is definitely not plumber crack." I'm sure that none of the high-spirited women pictured on the site decked out in New Year's Eve hats and a drink in hand would have ventured out on this adventure on her own. And none of them would have even researched the possibility of such a trip in a travel agent's office. Thanks to the Internet, they were able to go way off the reservation.

MATCHMAKING WILL NEVER BE THE SAME

Above all, the Internet has made more matches than all the Dolly Levis in history put together. I've heard countless stories of a long-lost love showing up within hours of establishing a

Facebook page. My cousin Mark found Meg, his college sweet-heart, whom he had rejected back then, because, as he now understands, he got frightened by the intensity of the relation-ship; he transferred to another school and did not see her for thirty years, during which time she got married and he got married twice. (After his second divorce he created Sudden-bachelor.com, a Web site for divorced men his age.) At the time they got back in touch, his second marriage was petering out. They chatted intensely and longingly for months, then arranged to meet. Soon after that, Meg, whose children were in college and whose marriage was also running out of steam, picked up and moved across the country to be with Mark. "He was always the love of my life," she said simply.

When my mother-in-law was widowed many years ago, she was in her fifties and hoping to find a second partner, but her only recourse was to show up at the Roseland Ballroom on a prescribed afternoon and dance for a couple of hours with other "middle-aged singles." The group didn't change very much—"the same old losers," she would report—but at least she got to dance, which she loved. (She ultimately met her second husband at work.) If she were around today, I am sure she would be scouring the Internet for a site that would specialize in unmarried people who, among other things, love to dance. Countless services—some very specialized—have made thousands of successful connections between people (roughly one-fourth of whom are over fifty) who most likely would have never met the old-fashioned way.

Mona has had personal experience with both. She did find her true love at midlife the old-fashioned way, but lightning would never have struck a second time if it weren't for the Internet. When she turned fifty, she counted her blessings. "Life is great," she told herself. "I've had great careers. I have wonderful friends. I have a great family. My parents were wonderful people. If I never meet anyone in my life, it's just not meant to be. This is a great life, and I'm going to live it the best I can." But, it turns out, finding love was meant to be.

Mona has a regular tennis doubles game, and one day, when one of the players didn't show up, someone asked Manuel, a portrait artist, to fill in. They hit it off. "It was the real thing for the first time," she says. "It was an incredible experience of being with someone who truly wanted to be with me as 'number one.' We traveled and we had fun and he was a lovely, kind man."

It is unlikely that a computerized analysis of interests and backgrounds would have made the match. Mona "was part of a nuclear family, third-generation American"; Manuel was one of eleven children in a close-knit Sephardic Jewish family that had emigrated from Morocco to France. His relatives were scattered all over the globe. "We traveled for every family event; the family was always together, and what that did is it gave me a sense of family and continuation that was absolutely different and foreign from what I had grown up with."

I hadn't noticed the past tense in her account until I asked where Manuel's studio was, and Mona responded, "He died." While she was nursing him through a long and painful bout of cancer, the far-flung family visited regularly and gave her enormous support. She continues to attend family occasions wherever they take place.

One year after Manuel's death, Mona was starting to get her life back together. Now that she had experienced the Real Thing, she didn't want to do without. "I said to myself, I have to find another Manuel." How on earth would she find another Moroccan-born French-speaking Sephardic Jew? Not on earth, but he was out there in cyberspace. It took a little ingenuity. She filled out the information profiles on a couple of online dating services, but to no avail. She kept trolling for new and offbeat sites; one was especially intriguing—it searched by specific words. She tried "Sephardic": nothing. Then she added "French-speaking."

Before she could check for replies, Mona left for Montreal and a concert some friends had invited her to. The headliner turned out to be a Sephardic singer from Tunisia. "It was a great concert. All the women who were over fifty were falling down, swooning," she recalls. When Mona got home, she checked the site where she had plugged in "French-speaking."

One of the three people who had replied, a widower, struck her fancy. God, he's cute, she thought to herself. He was also Jewish and from North Africa and had lived in France. Mona wrote back to "Recent widower": "I'm a recent widow. Just returned from the Sephardic music festival in Montreal . . . curious?" He replied, "What was an American woman doing at the Enrico Macias concert? Write or call?" She replied, "Write *and* call," and gave her phone number. Less than a year later, they moved in together. "We're going to take bike trips and do active things that neither of us could have done while we were caring for spouses who were very ill." In my most recent communiqué from her, she announced that they had eloped six months later.

Alice, who is sixty-one, does not believe in miracles. For her the Internet is a Chinese menu of sexual options. She sorts her online conquests into categories, and is very clear about what she wants from each of them. "I married for the second time at fifty-five to a man nineteen years older, who died three months later. We were together for six years, and the sex life was great! Since then I have met several men through online dating. I have had mind-blowing sex with three of them, one for love (who has an extremely low libido), and the other ones for sex only. I find that foreplay is more important than the act itself. My sensuality is just an extension of what it has been all my life, and I am not slowing down!"

Online dating has also produced a whole new set of

consumer pitfalls—"scams, players, liars," one woman complained. A British novelist named Charlotte Cory has turned her experiences as a fifty-year-old divorcée looking for love in cyberspace into a comic radio show called *Thinking of Leaving Your Husband?* She signed up for several matchmaking services. "And it was eye-opening," she told *The Times* of London. "As a novelist I thought I knew about human nature. I naïvely thought that when I met people I could gauge them, and what I discovered was that I knew nothing." She was totally unprepared for what she calls the "culture of dishonesty." "They send shifty-looking photographs, lie about their names, marital status, age." Ultimately, though, she did find the man for her. "There he was," she says of their first date, "my absolute perfect partner. He handed me his card; I read 'Professor Parrott' and nearly fell off my chair laughing. I said, 'If I marry you, I'm going to have to change my name to Polly.'" They did—and she did. Professor Parrott can't get over their good fortune and the alchemy the Internet is capable of. "We might have passed on the escalators, going opposite ways. Isn't it frightening that happiness should be so hit-and-miss?"

WHO SHALL I BE TODAY?

In the course of researching an art project online, Penny met a German businessman who had very similar interests. For eighteen months they corresponded daily—for hours. Penny would become so engrossed that once when a hurricane blew down a tree outside her window and crushed her car, she didn't even notice. Each of them wrote long, intimate, passionate e-mails, but she was always aware that despite the give-and-take and despite having exchanged photographs, it was "all happening in my head." The thoughts she was composing and the responses to his information, she cautioned herself, were being processed in her mind, not really between two present people. The relationship became intense and passionate in the Internet's titillating way.

Ultimately they arranged to meet—in Paris. They reserved a hotel room in the hopes that the meeting would go well. On the appointed day Penny was quivering with anticipation. When he appeared, the electricity between them was palpable and they spent a glorious day exploring the City of Love. Finally, they went back to the hotel. This is it! she thought. They kissed, and then he announced that he was totally impotent. And, what's more, he had no intention of seeking treatment. Penny was devastated; not only was the passion that their e-mails had stoked being squelched, but after all the truth telling and soul baring and falling in love, he had withheld a crucial piece of information. The relationship was indeed happening in her head, after all. She felt betrayed and rebuffed all his efforts to get back to how it was in cyberspace.

Michael Civin, who raises so many challenging questions about online intimacy, has an intriguing take on Internet duplicity. "Does the technology of cyberspace facilitate the emergence of alternative identities, of other ways of being human that otherwise remain trapped, encumbered, and dissociated?" he asks. "Does the emergence of cyberspace alter fundamentally the significance of gender, blending or socially mutating maleness and femaleness into techno-gendered email-ness?"

Joyce has created a pair of "alternative identities"—one that sleeps next to her uninterested husband and the other that frolics online—that for her add up to one full life. Before she found AshleyMadison.com, a dating site for married people, she felt she was leading half a life. At fifty she sold the business she had started, began to indulge her wander-lust in trips all over the world, and had a few affairs with men she met in her travels. Her husband of thirty-four years was older, more conservative, and traveled all the time for business; their sex life was nil. Considering her options, Joyce saw "three choices: one was to stay put and do absolutely nothing, and I wasn't going to do that, because it's not who I am; another was to get a divorce and find somebody that I could have a compatible sexual relationship with, but," she adds, "I was probably going to end up in the same boat." Besides, other than the sex, "my life was really good." She is very close to her two stepdaughters—"I was in the room when all my grandchildren were born," she recalls—and her hus-band, who is her "soul mate, bless his heart." So she chose the third option—"to figure out how to meet my physical and emotional needs in some other way."

The Internet provided the answer: access to like-minded married people who are interested in sex but have no intention of walking away from their family lives. Joyce has been meeting men that way for almost three years. Several of the relationships took place entirely online—they never met. If a lot of people are entirely satisfied by so-called "online cheating," have they created a new form of intimacy that raises the question: What, then, is the definition of "an affair"?

"I have met really interesting, intelligent, successful, well-intentioned gentlemen," Joyce tells me. One liaison lasted more than a year, "until his stepson used government surveillance software to hack into my computer and maliciously destroyed letters and photographs." But, she adds, "not even that stopped me. I went right back. There are lots of people out there who are just like me, who have everything going for them—they don't want to rock the boat." Most profess sexless marriages and "a chilly emotional state"; they are very clear about what they want, she explains. "Some are looking for just sex, some of them are looking for passion, some are looking for love." It gets even more specific. "There are little boxes on the site that you can check off—kissing, receiving oral sex, giving oral sex; you can check off threesomes. It just changes all the rules."

The opportunity to explore an alternative life on the Internet has taken Joyce to new realms of self-awareness. "I am discovering that I am an unconventional person and believe life offers us many opportunities for friendship and love and why be tied down to what is 'correct.'"

DO I DARE?

Historically, despite the waves of liberation, women who were drawn to the "incorrect," the kinky, the outrageous, repressed their desires or fulfilled them furtively. They were sure that if found out, they would be considered freaks or outcasts. No more. Like Joyce, who not only got in touch with her unconventional self in Second Adulthood but found affirmation in an Internet community of others, many women who have a lifetime of conventional behavior behind them are reveling in the discovery that they are not alone in their sexual curiosity. For them, the New Intimacy is about freedom and daring and honesty, as it is widely defined among them. Here are excerpts from a conversation about love after fifty on *More* magazine's Web site; the range of experience and the shameless—in the good sense—openness kept the freewheeling and highly civil conversation going for weeks:

> I love my husband of 13 years but I want to explore new relationships. I have a historical and social understanding of the history of marriage and I think it is still the best institution if you want to have children,

but other than that—it can be quite suffocating. Thank god I am a very strong powerful force not to get 'taken over' by my role as wife and mother—but for many years I left 'me' sitting on the shelf and now that I have re-discovered me, my mind and heart is open to new friendships. I have been most candid with my husband! Anyone else out there needing to stretch her wings?

After 21 years of marriage and 3 kids I am also interested in exploring the idea of open marriage. First up, how to introduce it to my husband?

It's probably the most nerve-wracking conversation you will ever have with him. In my experience, the only way was to 'just do it.' Be totally open and honest. And continue to assure him of your love. Talk, talk, talk . . . There are lots of websites and online groups . . . You are not alone.

I floated the idea out to my husband last night and now he's quiet. At least it has him thinking.

Would any of you consider bringing another woman into your marriage? Is the idea yucky? Would it cause additional problems for you, your husband or your third? Or do you feel like gay or bisexual means having partners of one gender at a time?

I have never been a jealous person—ever—all my life! This is one area that my husband struggled with—but after reading the poly sites and understanding the concept that it is possible to deeply love and care for more than one person he realized that it was not a threat to him or a reflection of him and our relationship.

I'm just wondering . . . don't you feel the slightest bit selfish?

Selfishness goes out the window in an open relationship. Depending on how many people you're involved with, you may be sharing yourself and them with several others. . . . Plus you aren't taking them from other people they love and who love them and they aren't taking you from people you love and who love you. This is about opening your self and your life to include other people who have come to mean so much to you that you can't imagine not having them in your life on an intimate basis.

I have a friend who gave this a try. She was single, but her guy was in an open marriage. They were crazy about each other. But over time she just couldn't take the sharing and always coming second to his long time wife. She thought she'd be OK with it but ultimately wasn't. AND she caught herpes from the guy on top of that.

I've done some exploring as a single midlife gal there's lots of interest out there in unconventional sex practices— LOTS. We have roots in the age of Aquarius, after all.

That may well be, but however kooky or unconventional we were back then, it is also true that *we are not who we were only older* now. If we are kooky or unconventional now, it is in terms we are defining for ourselves, not measuring against the prevailing norm. When it comes to how we connect and whom we connect with, all bets are off. The permeable membrane between the world we live in and cyberspace makes for wondrous and confusing emotional transmogrifications.

Technology has transformed the way we meet new people, share our secrets, make ourselves vulnerable, experience empathy, and even how we define *faithfulness*. It has also liberated our way of making ourselves known to one another: timid people don't have to test their courage face-to-face; people who are self-conscious about their looks can share what our mothers used to call "the beauty within." In the process, we may discover new aspects of our true selves and at the same time enter totally "other" personas, which we may or may not choose to bring back into the Real World.

Online communication expands the definition of *intimacy* and at the same time enables us to affirm profound expressions of love. For better and for worse—most would say for better—love, sex, and intimacy have forever changed in our lifetime.

Chapter 5

Love and Work—Together at Last

Love and work are the cornerstones of our humanness.

—Erik H. Erikson, *Childhood and Society*

Ours is the first generation of women to even imagine, let alone experience, loving their work. Although women have always earned what little they could in low-wage jobs, the workplace reforms of the sixties and seventies—opening up male-only job categories, establishing the principle of equal pay for equal work, developing antidiscrimination guidelines, and even beginning the stirrings of family-leave policies—released a wave of ambition and determination that carried women into the marketplace. Once there, we broke through sacred barriers (in 1975 a pundit told *Ms.* magazine that there would never be a woman news anchor in our lifetime, because "people just wouldn't take a female voice seriously") and established solid credentials. We began to be taken seriously and we built our collective power.

At the same time, a woman who worked outside the home was torn between the demands of work and the demands of family or love life. There was never enough self to go around, and many of us were tormented by the feeling that we were fulfilling neither relationship as well as we should have been. In an effort to economize on our resources, we often put our own needs, interests, and energy in third place, and although we were, in effect, doing two full-time jobs, we were supposed to be grateful for the opportunity to Have It All. It was almost impossible to integrate the two spheres, no matter how hard we tried. But we found that rewards from one could compensate for perceived failures in the other. Sometimes work saved us from problems with love. Sometimes love lost out to work. Sometimes work *was* love.

We are still remodeling the love-and-work component as we assemble the pieces of our lives for the next stage. And this time out, we have more room—more time, fewer responsibilities, more focus, less stress—to maneuver. For many women, establishing a New Intimacy with working will enrich their Second Adulthood's portion of connection, appreciation, community, affect, and joy.

LOVING YOUR DAY JOB

As we reach Second Adulthood, there are many women for whom work has had an important impact on their most intimate relationships; there are also many for whom work has been an intimate relationship in itself; and there are some for whom it has been the primary relationship. Each of us will approach the chance to realign her personal mix of worldly and spiritual commitment with a new set of dreams, frustrations, and burdens.

I have been one of the lucky ones who has loved her work, and also been blessed with other (mostly) supportive and nurturing human relationships at home. When my work is going well, the feeling is lovelike. I think about it even if I am doing other things; I get excited when I embark on a particularly interesting task; I lose track of time when I am engrossed in it; and when I was deprived of my work (fired), I felt totally bereft. I know that working on something—or working *at* something—that matters to me will continue to be an intimate part of who I am.

I also had the experience of being able to count on the emotional sustenance from a workplace community. I can recall times when it felt like the *only* emotional sustenance in my life. I still cherish the "Thank God It's Monday Club," formed with a couple of colleagues to celebrate the day in the week when we returned from a weekend of stress and chaos to a place where we felt competent and appreciated.

Maria has a similar connection to her job. Although she doesn't love her work—it is fairly routine and tedious—she loves going to work and has no intention of giving that up. She runs a small post office in eastern Pennsylvania. During her twenty-three years there, she has raised three children on her own and advanced on the job. She likes being good at what she does, but what she loves about her days is the constant interaction with the people in her community. "Knowing most of the folks who come into the post office means that I can keep up with their lives," she says. "And seeing familiar faces has raised my spirits on many occasions." Without that ingredient in her life, she says, "I would feel lost—and useless."

Teri, a fifty-eight-year-old fabric designer, is an extreme case. Art is and always has been her all-encompassing source of joy; it is clearly her most intimate relationship. "I would be a very difficult person to live with; it would take an extraordinary person to put up with my saying things like 'Sorry, I need to go knit.'" There are, of course, loving relationships in her life. One friend lives down the hall—they touch base several times a day—and others will show up "at the drop of a hat," if needed. "I treasure my friends," she says. "I absolutely treasure them." But despite the fact that it barely pays her bills, the most important relationship in her life is, she says, "my work and making art! For me making art means whether I am painting or knitting or making jewelry, I have to force myself to take a breath and sit still."

Teri's life choice reflects the degree to which a commitment to a meaningful project—paid or not—can energize a woman's life at any stage. Good work is simply good for our well-being. Studies have shown that women with what neuropsychiatrist Louann Brizendine calls "high career momentum" scored higher "on measures of self-acceptance, independence, and effective functioning in their fifties and sixties, and rated their physical health higher than did other women." Moreover, even if the job itself leaves much to be desired, the workplace provides the kind of social network that is empowering and, the experts tell us, essential to healthy aging. As our families disperse, and our social life becomes more selective, the interaction with colleagues may be as good a reason as the paycheck to keep working, revise our work life, or enter the workforce at last.

The only conditions under which work has been shown to be *not* good for our well-being are when the worker feels she has no control over what she is doing and gets no recognition for her efforts. It is no coincidence that the same toxic conditions poison love as well. And it is not surprising that now that we have a chance to review the bidding, we are pushing for power sharing and respect in both our private and our public lives and working toward a healthy interdependence between them.

FROM TRADE-OFFS TO BALANCE

When we first entered the workforce in significant numbers, the push-back from the outside world was intense, but as we persevered, our own self-image was transformed. The fact that some women were making their way in the "man's world" changed the way we valued our skills, and that growing self-confidence affected what we were looking for in a partner. It became less necessary to look for a good provider or a source of reflected status. If we could pay our own way, we could make our own way. We could "become the men we wanted to marry."

Which did not mean that we didn't want to get married. Theoretically our financial independence would open up the field beyond that goal of "a good provider." As it turned out, even though the field of candidates was expanding to include prospects that no longer had to be taller, richer, better-educated, and more successful, it was also contracting by eliminating those men who didn't care for "uppity women" and "castrating bitches." These unfamiliar forces often threw us off-kilter. While many women established loving and nurturing relationships, others made misconceived choices and brutal trade-offs. Ironically, those who chose to go the traditional route found to their dismay that the job of wife and mother had been demeaned by the glorification of work "outside the home," as it was delicately called. Still others found the whole business too confusing and often demoralizing; they opted out by making the decision to commit to one and abandon the other.

The women who chose to marry and stay in the workplace soon found that the men they married had little ambition to become the women *they* wanted to marry, so we were left doing two jobs—"bring[ing] home the bacon," as the 1970s commercial for Enjoli perfume celebrated it, "and fry[ing] it up in the pan." The ad might extol the virtues of double duties in order to sell perfume, but at the same time, "experts" and "advisers" were warning that the stress generated by attempting the balancing act would take a toll on our health and even, it was argued, our fertility. What a price to pay!

It turns out, though, that for women trying to do two jobs, the stress came *after* work. Marianne Legato, an expert in gender-based medicine (which focuses on the particular characteristics of female physiology), cites a study of working couples in Sweden, which found that "when men and women arrived home, women's blood pressure and heart rates rose as they crossed the threshold, while men's fell!" Those once stressed-out women are arriving at a point in their lives where the pressure of their two jobs is abating, but the rewards of participating in the public sphere are still attainable.

The same is true for those who have made the opposite trade-off and opted to put work first. Women who have set aside other satisfactions to devote themselves to their careers can now focus on personal connections. A recent notice in an alumni magazine put it succinctly: "I've had the education (Harvard, Stanford, Wharton), rewarding careers (health care, higher ed), great locations (Boston area, currently Seattle). Now would love to get this relationship thing right. . . ."

Vivian Gornick, whose devotion to writing was more successful than any long-term relationships, looks back on her single life with mixed emotions. "No choice was ever without serious contradictions or regret on my part," she writes, but she also celebrates her hard-won agency in the world of success and impact; she treasures the "privilege" of being a woman who is "living out the conflicts rather than the fantasies." Like many others who took the career path, she has no children.

Martha devoted her first adulthood to a sales job she loved. She had many friends, but because she traveled so much while most of them were establishing families, she drifted away from their day-to-day lives. Her setup precluded forming any serious love relationships, which, she now realizes, was just the way she wanted it. She came from a very unhappy family and feared becoming vulnerable; she also did not want to have children. Work gave her everything she needed, including protection from getting involved.

When she was approaching her fiftieth birthday and also entering menopause, though, Martha found herself taking stock, and, typically, became restless with her life as it was.

"I didn't want to be work-defined anymore." She cut back on her traveling, concentrated on reacquainting herself with old friends and making some new ones who "were not as professionally successful," and even reluctantly accepted a few blind dates.

Within a few years, she met and married a widower. "He made me feel safe," she explains. They were very much in love, but found it extremely difficult to reconcile their two past lives—her total independence and his traditional domesticity. His extended family embraced Martha and gave her the kind of warmth she had missed; his son, whom he doted on—indulged was the way she saw it—was more of a problem. As they merged their lives, the question was, in Martha's words, "How do two people who are used to making decisions come together and make joint decisions?" She was also disconcerted by the realization that while she was no longer a workaholic, she was now married to one. So, in addition to preserving their independence, they needed to start from scratch to create a zone of interdependence. They set up "date nights" and found a language for communicating what each needed from the other—and when. Martha has totally shifted gears, though she still does consulting in her field, for this new love-oriented chapter of her life, which she is finding as satisfying as it is different from the work-oriented years.

For some professionally focused women, the shift is taking place within their work experience. The drive to get ahead is giving way to the notion that work with meaning has more appeal than work with perks. Essayist Anna Quindlen, who has come to that point herself, suggests redefining the measure of success by "satisfaction of the spirit, rather than by power of the résumé." For someone who has spent a lifetime on the fast track, the switch can reveal a local stop that offers an array of intriguing sights and sounds.

That understanding is behind a growing movement toward "encore careers"—paid jobs that utilize and build upon the skills we have already accumulated in our work life and apply them in the service of societal, rather than purely commercial, needs; "trading money for meaning," as Marc Freedman has put it. In his new book, *The Big Shift: Navigating the New Stage Beyond Midlife,* Freedman quotes a woman who had been working happily in a corporate job until the company was shut down. In the course of the following "year of reflection"—her Fertile Void—she had a revelation. "I couldn't do another corporate job. . . . I'm a product of the sixties, for crying out loud," she said. "I need to feel passionate about my work. I need to do something that makes me cry, for good reasons, and I hadn't felt that kind of commitment or passion about a job for years and years." She now runs Crossroads, the largest homeless service organization in Rhode Island; she loves the work but does not love the struggle to get by on her diminished income.

MAKING WORK AND LOVE WORK

At midlife it is possible—but not easy—to create a healthy *interdependence* of work, love, and personal fulfillment—essential ingredients, which poet and author David Whyte aptly identifies as "marriages." "Everyone is committed, consciously or unconsciously, to three marriages," he writes. "There is the first marriage, the one we usually mean, to another; that second marriage, which can so often seem like a burden, to a work or vocation; and that third and most likely hidden marriage to a core conversation inside ourselves." They are inseparable and not interchangeable; one can't be traded away to make room for another. "To neglect any one of the three is to impoverish them all, because they are not actually separate commitments but different expressions of the way each individual belongs to the world." Each of those marriages can become an expression of the New Intimacy. Together they can make life in Second Adulthood add up to more than the sum of its parts.

We each arrive at this stage of life with our own set of conflicts about love, work, and our needs. But resources we developed along the way are emboldening us to change and reconfigure all three marriages. Each comes with its own challenges.

The first marriage may require the most immediate attention. Any transition in the life of either partner destabilizes the existing balance—or imbalance—of power. If, for example, one person has been calling the shots, what happens if the game changes? If the financial contribution of one partner goes up or down, how does that affect the domestic setup? Who takes out the garbage? What's next?

And if both are going through a major transition—typically, the emptying of the family nest—the challenges are compounded. Though many find that rite of passage less traumatic than advertised (not unlike the situation with menopause), couples still need to reacquaint themselves with each other as people rather than as parents.

Cindy and her husband of forty years had moved to Toronto to raise their children in an environment where they could pursue their careers and still maintain a close-knit family life. Their stable life became unbalanced when their children moved to a city a thousand miles away and their grandchildren were born there. Things got even more off-kilter when Ed was diagnosed with non-Hodgkin's lymphoma and had to undergo a lengthy regimen of chemotherapy. His illness focused Cindy's attention on the preciousness of their marriage—his devotion as a father and supportive love as a partner—which she had taken for granted.

As she approached sixty, the mainstays of Cindy's life were changing. While her work was still challenging and rewarding, everything else had shifted; the intimacy that had revolved around her children was running down, while the desire to bond with her grandchildren was heating up and her husband's illness had awakened her to the fragility of their time together. Ed's world was in flux also; he worried about his health, was anxious to get back to work—and missed the grandchildren. Together they decided to turn the page by moving to where their children and grandchildren were, so they could become involved in their daily lives, and where they would try to reestablish themselves professionally and socially. After two years, they have both found work that is meaningful, but not as intense as in the past, and have reinvented the family life—including their marriage— that had been so important in their first adulthood.

"DON'T RETIRE, REWIRE"

Cindy and Ed haven't retired; they have reoriented their priorities significantly, but they are still doing work that matters to them. What happens when the work piece—no matter how unrewarding—is set aside altogether? How do people fill the void? Retirement, we are told, should be "at least as much fun as fourth grade," but it can be tricky getting to the fun part when there is so much at stake. If you are on your own, the prospect of filling your days with activities and relationships and your bank account with a safety net can be daunting, to say the least. If you have a partner, you may be stunned by her or his totally different vision. Travel or stay home and read the great books. Volunteer or play tennis. Join the peace corps or the local amateur theater. Move to someplace warm or move to be near the grandchildren. Differences about budgeting money, how to deal with extended family, and how to allocate time—alone, with friends, pursuing interests, with each other—can't be avoided. Any interdependence that has been established so far in the marriage will have to be renegotiated. Which is not necessarily a bad thing.

A cottage industry in weekend retreats has sprung up to help couples articulate and address their feelings about work now and in the future, their marriage, and any dreams they have for themselves as well as any sense of loss (the empty nest, career, physical capacity) at this stage of life. Many people—especially men—have told me they found that the experience refreshed their marriage. They are glad, they usually add, that their wives "made" them do it. Most women don't think they need a formal setup to figure out what they feel (just a good lunch with the girls) or what needs to change in the marriage going forward (she's kept a running list for the last twenty years). But if she is contemplating making changes, she's going to have to deal with his—perhaps surprising—expectations for himself and their life together, so she would do well to encourage him to spell them out. Even if they are both on the same page, there may be unexpected challenges to their work/family equation.

One of the biggest complaints from women whose partners have retired is that she becomes his only source of intimacy ("I married him for better or for worse, but not for lunch" is a familiar cry), whereas even if she has retired too, she has her circle of trust. As one woman told the authors of *Smart Women Don't Retire—They Break Free,* "Four of the most dreaded words to a wife are 'I'll go with you.'" In whatever form of New Intimacy a couple works out, time apart will be as important to preserve as time together used to be. "Marriage," wrote John Updike in *Gertrude and Claudius,* "must flow through intervals of privacy; otherwise a sludge of resentments never has time to clear." Rae attributes the success of her new relationship to a remix of work and love. "I don't know whether it's love or like," she says, "but I enjoy being with him, in bed and out. An important bond is the fact that we both work—he is seventy-five and works two days a week, while I, at seventy-three, write freelance and teach. And we both adore our grandchildren."

The word *retire* is distressing for most of us, even if we are trying to diminish our workload. Perhaps because we associate it with "shy and retiring," the traditional female attributes that, now more than ever, we have no truck with. The last thing we feel like doing is pulling back from life, yet it is rarely clear where to go next. Jeri Sedlar and Rick Miners have captured the spirit of reinvention in the title of their very helpful book *Don't Retire—Rewire!* Rewiring our relationship to the world at large calls for some risk taking and some compromises as well.

THE OTHER MARRIAGE—WORK

After taking into account finances and opportunities, some women are revising their marriages to work by striking out on their own. Luckily we have become risk takers with age and have less sensitivity to what other people think of our choices. So we can move on from foolish ideas and bounce back from failures before hitting our stride—starting a business that fizzles and then one that succeeds; retiring and then changing our mind; going to school to get training in a job it turns out we are no good at. Some may give up; others may find their courage rekindled at every stage.

Donna Edwards, now a respected congresswoman from Maryland, was close to fifty, working in an organization and just out of a bad marriage, when she took the plunge. "I was very unhappy with the person who was a seven-term incumbent," she says but "if I had stayed in that marriage I would never be in Congress now." When she began to think about running, "Just about everyone I talked to said, 'Don't do it.'" She didn't take their advice. "Very quietly one Friday before Easter, I drove to Annapolis and I filled out the form and I wrote my check for a hundred dollars and I went home and didn't tell anybody." Finally she began to campaign—without the support of the skeptics who said "it was ridiculous and insane." She lost that election "by a couple of hundred votes—actually 2,731 votes." But she dusted herself off and ran again. This time she got more support and won. "It was a huge risk doing something I'd never done before," she recalls. "But it was all so freeing and liberating."

Volunteering—as ticklish a word as *retirement*—can be a training ground for new ventures. Long-standing community commitments may have become more compelling with time; or it may be possible to explore a whim by volunteering in a related field. A doctor in California has closed her practice and works two days a week in a local clinic. (She has found the need so great that she has enticed some former colleagues to sign up too.)

Taking courses (with or without credit) to update skills or simply to stimulate those "little gray cells" is an increasingly appealing option for older students, as educational institutions become more welcoming to them. I know a retired banker who is studying the history of textiles. (She is spreading the two-year course over three so she "can have a life," which, she observes, her younger classmates don't seem to have.) A former actress considered her love of animals and her commitment to feminism and found that she could combine them by taking a seminar in sociobiology. A hobby or an aptitude that has been taken for granted may look different from a more relaxed perspective. It may even awaken an entrepreneurial spirit: A weekend Ms. Fix-It in Cleveland got some professional training and has opened a small contracting business.

When I read about one truly offbeat lifestyle choice, I was

delighted to find an example of a midlife change that literally takes those who embrace it off the reservation. Even better, it represents a very innovative example of how the many "retirement" considerations can be accommodated at once in a newly reconfigured setup. It's not just about income or adventure or finding a new community or downsizing—or shocking the kids, which it often does—but about a serious makeover that combines all of the above. In a little heralded and increasingly popular "work camper" program, an estimated eighty thousand semiretired vagabonds travel from national park to national park in their RVs, earning a small salary in exchange for hours spent doing everything from leading nature walks to picking up trash. Especially in these hard economic times, their efforts play a vital role in keeping park life going, even, in some cases, keeping the parks open.

Most are attracted to the roving life during a reassessment period after some midlife upheaval, and many have been delighted to find that they can find community (even, in a few cases, love) and continue to pursue and develop their interests. One, a retired biologist who lives alone in her trailer, leads bird-watching walks. A former nurse guides canoe trips down the Rio Grande for groups interested in nature. When they move on, the campers stay in touch by e-mail, and usually meet up again further down the road.

When contemplating retirement, there seems to be a pervasive disconnect between how women—who have for the most part held back during the family years—and men—who want to get off the treadmill—view the importance of work in their future plans. When she announced her retirement from an accounting firm, Sara was surprised to discover a male-female dichotomy in the reactions. The men had two concerns, which they expressed in sober tones: "Are you sick?" and "What are you going to *do*?" The women almost universally expressed enthusiasm: "That's wonderful; just don't rush into anything right away. Enjoy your freedom first." Which is exactly the way she sees it. She is looking forward to exploring the possibilities that she knows await her.

FINDING A PASSION—OR A PILOT LIGHT

One of the reasons that a man may be burned out while a woman is rarin' to go is that most of us have taken a circuitous route—regretfully bypassing some options—to our current work situation, while most men have proceeded along a fairly straight trajectory. For a woman who is renegotiating a long-running relationship with a burned-out partner at the same time that she is fired up to make some changes in her work life, the future looks especially confusing. Both seem to call for a kind of rekindled passion. But what if nothing takes fire? One of the pervasive myths of the transition to the rest of our lives is that only a driving passion will light the way—in both love and work.

A few of us do have a driving passion, but even fewer were able to follow it earlier on. For those lucky few, this may be a time to go for it—with single-minded and audacious zeal. During most of her adult life Cara never left home without her camera in hand; stunning black-and-white photographs of animals and landscapes hang throughout the rambling farmhouse in which she and her husband, Will, have raised their two children. Throughout the same thirty years, Cara and Will have worked hard building a business in handicrafts, often at great sacrifice. They are a close family, have lots of friends, and love to entertain, but Christmas is their business's busiest time and they have often had to give the holidays very short shrift.

Recently, though, their son has gone into the business and Cara has been able to spend more time pursuing her passion. The love of photography has moved on to making documentaries. Using digital equipment that was unheard-of earlier, she has recently completed an eighteen-month project, filming the daily life of a local organic farmer. She has never been happier and holidays are warm and full of life at last.

Most of us, though, don't come up with an identifiable burning passion, no matter how hard we look for it. Then we berate ourselves for not finding it. The truth is that most of us aren't built that way. Barbara didn't set out with a vision; she was pushed. When she was let go from her HR job, she was shocked and panicky. "Now what?" she asked herself, but she was unable to think ahead. Her sisters had both moved to California years earlier and had been urging her to join them. As she had nothing to lose, Barbara put her possessions in storage, packed up her car, and . . . couldn't get out of her driveway. After sitting paralyzed in her idling car for a time, she made a couple of desperate phone calls to friends and family; finally, with their reassurance, she got going—with a "sense of real courage." It was no easier to reestablish herself professionally on the West Coast than it had been back East. Then she was "hit with a blinding flash of the obvious." A longtime conservationist, she harnessed that hobby (she would never call it a passion) and combined it with her professional skill into a totally new job description—"'green career coaching,' specializing in career tracks in a green market sector or industry." That was in 2004; the business is thriving and she calls it her "dream job."

The lesson we have learned about fairy-tale love stories applies equally to the notion of unearthing a long-lost dream project when we finally have the chance. We ultimately discover that in work, as in true love, our guiding lights are not fireworks but "pilot lights"—low-intensity, but always on. They do not consume us, but they light the way ahead.

The longing for an undefined passion is related to a chronic deficiency many of us bring to this moment—no real game plan for ourselves. We have plenty of experience in dreaming about finding true love, but little experience in constructing practical dreams of our own. When love overshadows all other aspirations, a woman's life becomes a precarious series of contingencies: If he does X, then I will try to do Y, but if that changes or I have kids, I will have to try Z, and if he leaves me, I will be forced to do XYZ.

We all know of a woman who postponed her education to put her husband through school, or one who turned down a promotion because it would require longer hours, or one who was just about to open her own shop when her husband's job required the family to move, or one who had just embarked on some professional training when her husband left her. Those women couldn't count on being able to stick with any project, let alone a long-term plan. When it is finally possible for them to consider what they have always wanted to do and pursue those goals, many women find they have none.

Psychiatrist Anna Fels has seen countless women who can't build a future of their own in the outside world because they have never let themselves imagine it. When she asked women—even young women, who have more encouragement to be ambitious than our generation did—about their plans,

Fels got "wildly diverse scenarios" with dramatically diverse psychological consequences, she reports in *Necessary Dreams: Ambition in Women's Changing Lives*. Some of the descriptions were vivid and promising, but many were vague and random—either "overly ambitious and unachievable at one extreme or uninspiring and unchallenging on the other." Fels observes further, "The more diffuse or undeveloped the story, the more anxious or joyless was the person sitting across from me," whereas "the liveliness and pleasure with which the women told their stories often corresponded closely to their level of self-esteem and general sense of well-being." We need to learn more, she concludes, about the "process by which women create, realize, reconfigure, and abandon goals." We are in the midst of doing just that in terms of both love and work.

Eileen's work history is familiar in its reactive randomness. She grew up in California and went to college there. "I didn't take courses with a career in mind," she realizes, looking back. "I took them to improve myself, to make myself more interesting." She worked briefly at a clerical job and then spent more than a year on her own in Europe. Soon after she got back, she met her husband. He had a daughter from his first marriage who had some physical problems that took a lot of attention; then Eileen gave birth to their own daughter. She stayed at home to care for her children.

"It seemed the natural order of things," she explains. "Most of my friends were stay-at-home moms."

After eight years, the demands at home let up a bit, and Eileen got a part-time job at a travel agency, which reconnected her with an earlier interest; "I always loved to travel, so that was perfect." The paycheck, as small as it was, gave her the self-esteem and financial wherewithal to think about going back to another abandoned interest. "I had always wanted to get a degree," she admits, but her husband was skeptical. She took another clerical job to cover her tuition and graduated with a degree in psychology when she was forty-four years old. Insecure as she still was, she had the fortitude to set herself up as (of all things) a career counselor. But she didn't dare commit; by the time her daughters were out of the house, she had three part-time jobs.

Then what happened? "Menopause," she explains. "I went through a metamorphosis in midlife. I think a lot of women homemakers live vicariously. You are in a support role. Suddenly I wanted my turn. I don't know what it is, but I'm drawn to wanting to get out there. Something I've got to do right now." Fertile Void confusion generated ideas all over the place. Her growing courage and energy took her from one to another until she clicked in.

First up was the very risky prospect of writing a book about boomer women. She spent several years doing research, but couldn't focus on it or sell the idea to a publisher. "My dreams were dashed," she says, but that effort led to the next, which was where her impulse to "get out there" took shape. "Looking back, it was one of the best things, because that was when I started my blog and my radio show." A friend who had been following Julie Powell's online chronicle of her journey through every recipe in Julia Childs's cookbook (it later became the hit movie *Julie and Julia*) suggested that Eileen try blogging (yet another option created by the Internet). Why not? she thought to herself. Her Web site, addressed to women her age, attracted a following and connected her with a woman who had a blog talk-radio show; that sounded like fun too, so she went for her own show. Feisty Side of Fifty—a site for "an amazing and bodacious group of women who are reinventing the spirit and style of aging"—is thriving.

Writing on her blog about the chapter of her life in which she took charge of her "turn," she contrives a mysterious love affair. "I was in my midforties when the affair began," she explains. "Interestingly, it was with someone whose value I'd discounted for many years. Though this isn't in my nature, I openly derided her (yes, it is a woman), smirking and pointing out her physical flaws to my friends. I even called her 'stupid'—something I never do. She just didn't seem the caliber person I could admire in the way I had so many others in my life." Eileen came around, though, she writes. "She had a lovely smile and a generous nature" and "was rather intelligent and had several gifts I'd never noticed before. In fact, I made a point of telling her how much I loved her and appreciated her body, mind, and soul." Who is this mysterious stranger? "My Self." Not surprisingly, she has found, as she fell in love with her Self and established her worth in the world, that her husband has come to appreciate her and respect her more as well, and that her "three marriages" are finally in order.

Shelly is not a risk taker like Eileen, but she too has found an equilibrium. The impulse that bubbled up around the time she turned fifty was to "re-create myself a little bit." That was risky enough. Until then she had nourished a successful corporate career with extensive travel and high-stress office politics, an active social life (no "emotional entanglements" but lots of ballroom dancing), and a twenty-year commitment to mentoring young women. The pieces were all there, but she felt the need to retool them. Re-creating her work took her from corporate work to running a small and dedicated not-for-profit organization that helps women make the kind of transition she has made. She also moved on from ballroom dancing to marriage.

The one piece that didn't change was her commitment to her mentees—and theirs to her. "I certainly have become a very trusted person in their lives," Shelly says. "Right now one of the young women is having marital problems and she can't talk to her parents about it, and she can't talk to people at work, and she isn't talking to her friends about it; I think I'm

really the one person, since I've known her husband as well."
Shelly has just taken on her twelfth mentee. She invited all of
them to her fiftieth birthday party, which included her
extended intimate circle of friends and family, and most
came. "That meant a lot to me," she says. For Shelly, a more
personal connection to her work—her first marriage—and a
loving relationship with her husband—her second—combine
with the long-standing intimacy she has established with the
next generation to make for a rewarding marriage between
herself and what matters to her.

THE CHANGES AROUND US AND WITHIN US

At the same time that we are reviewing our love and work
lives, we have to deal with changes taking place around us
and how they can undermine our self-esteem and challenge
our resourcefulness—the marriage with Self. Economic crises,
outdated skills, and ageism pure and simple are major factors. Essayist Kennedy Fraser is especially clear-eyed about a
common and subtle penalty of becoming an older woman
worker. "A man of my own age, with whom I was talking at
a party, withdrew his attention from me to look hungrily at a
pretty young woman many years my junior. As a young
woman I had relied on the attention of older men and
depended on their approval. I saw very clearly at that instant
when the man's gaze shifted that one kind of power had

passed from me. The time had come," she concluded wisely, "to develop other resources" for maintaining her effectiveness in the world. Those new resources may just turn out to feel more comfortable and authentic than earlier styles.

Tina, a CEO, also realized that until her late fifties, "my sexuality has always come into play in the power relationships I've had." She had developed an effective nonconfrontational technique "to deal with all the alpha males in my life; I'd circumvent them in various ways." Looking back, she realizes that the strategy of seduction and subterfuge "did not make for a very healthy relationship." When she changed her tactics and began to stand up to those same men, she confirmed the experience many of us have had: that saying no does not bring down the whole edifice—and often consumes a lot less time and energy than working under the radar. At first she was sure she "would lose. But actually I hardly ever did." And how did they respond? Ironically, instead of bullying, "*they* started going underground," practicing their version of subterfuge and devious methods, which were tactics she was well equipped to recognize and manipulate right back.

Joanne's story falls into three distinct chapters, each devoted to working out one of the "marriages." Not until she was sixty did the pieces of her life that had been estranged come together. For most of her first adulthood, work was the only thing that worked—a steady source of satisfaction and financial reward. Love was a series of operatic disasters. And Self, she realizes now, was an unknown quantity. Looking back on her early adulthood in the sixties and seventies, she recalls, "I partied all night, and the kind of men I was attracted to were all 'bad boys.'" By the time she got married briefly at thirty-two, she had already lived with five men. The marriage lasted eight years, and she lived with the next guy for nine. "I was sequentially monogamous," she says. Throughout all those relationships, she remained "detached." The saving grace was her day job. "I was secure in my work and used my work as a way to avoid intimacy."

When menopause hit, Joanne went into a tailspin that took her into a black hole. "It made me confused in my body. I became incredibly insecure," she says. As she wandered her Fertile Void, she found the will to make some changes: She ended her relationship, and for the first time in her life she lived alone—no man in her life. She loved her newfound privacy and didn't miss sex. Her friends and her career—and an Abyssinian cat she acquired—filled her life. "I was so happy!" she says. For two years she spent quality time alone with herself considering her resources.

By the time John came along, she was ready to make more life-affirming choices. This time she didn't run away from intimacy, and she found it with a totally unfamiliar breed of man for her—eight years younger, two children (she has none), "short, nerdy, glasses, and, of all things, a Republican." (On their first date they fought furiously about politics. "For some reason my ability to just explode in rage at this man was like a liberation of sorts.") But, she adds, "He's smart, he's thoughtful, and he's fearless and has an astonishing resilience." And one more thing, unlike every previous man she was attracted to, he's not "looking to me to save him."

"I have never felt more fulfilled than I feel at this moment," Joanne says. She just received a major promotion. "I feel like I have the exact right job that I've been waiting for without knowing it." And John is the partner she was waiting for "without knowing it." "He's a man who was completely, totally ill suited to me. I wouldn't have looked twice at him in the past," she says. "He makes me laugh—he's funny, we laugh in bed all the time. And I love to be with him. It's astonishing to me." They have been together for two years. He has just moved in. Stay tuned.

Joanne sees this convergence of love and work in her life in historical context. "I never thought I could change so much! I never thought such fulfillment was going to be possible. Our generation has been through an extraordinary thing. We've passed through being goosed in the hall, being in every way second-class citizens. We've watched everything change and have lived through it and have reached this stage—we've passed through it all and can come to this peaceful place; it's a great thing."

A "peaceful place" is not a resting place—the balancing

act goes on—but a state of mind; it is the place where the conflicts between love and work can be reconciled, where the sense of mastery that we have achieved is acknowledged, and where the capacity for creating a new kind of mutual and interdependent intimacy with other people is celebrated. Where—to use Erikson's word—we embrace our "humanness."

Chapter 6

The Child Within Grows Up

Oh the comfort, the inexpressible comfort of feeling
safe with a person, having neither to weigh thoughts nor
measure words, but pouring them all right out, just as they
are—chaff and grain together—certain that a faithful hand
will take and sift them, keeping what is worth keeping, and
with the breath of kindness blow the rest away.

—Dinah Maria (Mulock) Craik, "A Life for a Life" (1859)

Ruthie and I were best friends from grade school through
high school. I have an indelible image of the two of us sitting
cross-legged on the floor of her family's sun porch playing a
card game called Russian bank for hours on end. We had
twin families, we thought: European fathers; upbeat, somewhat flirty mothers (who, unlike other parents, took piano

lessons); and pesky little brothers. We even lived in similar houses in the same neighborhood. Over the years we were reassured by our shared circumstances and marveled at our synchronicity. One frigid winter weekend, our families went skiing for the first and only time. That was in the days of wooden skis, lace-up boots, and itchy woolen ski pants. On the first day out, I was cold and wet and scared and wanted to go back to the hotel. When we finally did, Ruthie and I discovered that we both had frozen our toes; we also confessed to each other that we had wet our pants. How's that for a bonding experience!

After high school, though, we went our separate ways—to different colleges and different lives. She married, had three children, and lived in the Midwest; I went across the country to start my career. Occasionally I would hear about her—that she had moved abroad with her husband and then that she had divorced him and was living with her children in Washington, D.C. In the meantime, I had moved back to New York, worked at a series of magazine jobs, married, and held off having children for fifteen years.

When I was writing *Inventing the Rest of Our Lives,* a former classmate told me that Ruthie had become a therapist and was leading groups for women, called "Retirement—or What Next," that dealt with the same issues of transition and turmoil and self-doubt that I was writing about. We made a date to visit, and it was as if we had played Russian bank the day before, not thirty years ago. We talked and talked, the way reunited lovers do, and seamlessly reentered each other's lives.

The parallels have continued in the years since then. Just after we reconnected, Ruthie's pesky brother died prematurely; mine had died in the eighties. Our mothers still lived on in the houses we had grown up in and were both still taking piano lessons. In recent months both declined, and a few months ago her mother died. Taking a break from the dreary business of closing up the house her family had lived in for more than sixty years, she brought me up to date on the dismantling process in a sort of free-verse e-mail that began:

> Understanding more and more about Mom; her personality; her history; what she saved; how she saved; how much she did for us; how much she left for me to do now.
>
> The tedium of the work.
>
> The enormity of the job
>
> The surprises unfolding.
>
> Many thoughts about saving/holding on to so much to such an extent for so long.
>
> A life.
>
> Death.
>
> Intensity.

Reading her words, I see her mom, I see the house, I see the clutter and know a similar scene awaits me.

People we grew up with—friends, or childhood sweethearts, or a particularly influential adult—have a special relationship with who we have become. Even if they haven't been in our peripatetic lives for years. That may be why as we engage in the process of inventing the rest of our lives, we reconnect and even search for each other. "We grew up together"; "She was my high school basketball coach"; "We shared a room in college"; "He was my first boyfriend"; "We've been through a lot together." Whether embracing or troublesome, those relationships are embedded in our personal narratives. They knew us back before we defined ourselves, and they defined intimacy for us before any others.

When lifelong friendships like Ruthie's and mine are established in childhood, the friends have yet to construct the barriers and boundaries that we all develop to protect ourselves. The history of one is preserved in the amber of the other's own childhood recollections. Even when the level of intimacy is more superficial, the transparency of our daily lives gives grade-school friends special access to each other's private experiences. We remember each other's parents, and had probably overheard them arguing on at least one occasion; we have a clear picture of each other's rooms. That is why when we meet at reunions, we marvel at how quickly we reconnect—recalling meaningful moments and rekindling casual familiarity. All the living in between melts away, and after a few minutes of reminiscing, we look to each other exactly the way we did when we first met.

It's also fascinating to see how those unformed characters turned out and contemplate how our own history might have been foreseen by those who knew us then. "One of my former classmates has a lot of money these days, and he moves in some very powerful circles," says Fran. "Nobody would have ever pointed at this particular guy and said, 'Oh, yes he'll be this type of person.' And yet when I see him now I think, Oh, I can see it—I can see the things in him now, I saw them then, but I just didn't recognize them then."

While those preadult friendships were volatile and often took on operatic proportions, the connection we established with classmates was an island in the storm of adolescent confusion. "In that critical period we attach to friends and peers almost as if they were blood relations," says psychoanalyst Colleen Konheim. "Those connections, those friendships made between the ages of fourteen and twenty-five, are often the strongest we make in our lives."

It is in those relationships that we learn about intimacy— how to listen and empathize, how to fight and make up. "No one can teach you what a great friend is, what a fair-weather friend is, what a treacherous and betraying friend is, except to have a great friend, a fair-weather friend, or a treacherous and betraying friend," says psychologist Michael Thompson, author of *Best Friends, Worst Enemies: Understanding the Social Lives of Children*. At my high school reunion, someone proposed a toast "to the fact that when we were twelve years old, we made some pretty good decisions about people." Everyone applauded.

"We love each other," says Fran of her group of five friends from high school who have maintained a continuous history with one another that many of us envy. "We talk all the time, and we've always made it a priority to get together regularly," she says. "When our kids were small it was just once a year, and now it's more like six or seven times a year; we go on vacation together, do things. Believe me," she goes on, "we are not all perfect, that's for sure; there have been aggravating moments along the way, but really you just don't have anybody who you can be as open about a lot of stuff as you are with friends like that."

Hers is an unusual lifelong circle of trust. They have been through marriages, divorces, children, financial crises, upheavals of all sorts—together. Nowadays, as they approach their sixties, they are encountering an even deeper level of intimacy—confronting death together. "One of my friends has cancer now and is going through a really rough time," says Fran sadly, "so we go down to her house in Florida; we bring food and we all hang out with her, and she cheers up." What is most amazing about this experience, she adds, is that the women are still encountering unexpected resources in one another. "I don't quite understand it—she soldiers on, and she's kept herself very stress-free; this was a woman who worried about everything, *everything*! So it's kind of a miracle, because she has kind of like done a complete reversal of her way of operating."

A measure of how deep such roots go is how painful it is when they are torn up. "The story of a breakup with a friend often feels far more revealing than that of a failed romance, as if it exposes our worst failings and weaknesses," write the authors of a book about the subject, called *The Friend Who Got Away*. "After all, an ex-friend is someone who knew our deepest secrets and then vanished, someone we drove away or who chose to leave us."

Those ruptures are stored away in private pockets of pain that are unsealed in the process of reviewing our lives. The desire to mend fences has sent many to the Internet in search of those lost friends. Not always with the desired result. I went to a recent reunion with a specific assignment: to find out why a former boyfriend has rebuffed my efforts over the years to get together and compare notes on our lives, the way old schoolmates do. I saw him walk in and confronted him. His reply was most unsatisfactory. "Those things happen," he said, and walked away. I will never know what it was that happened.

SOMETHING OLD AND SOMETHING NEW

The combination of preserved childhood vulnerability and grown-up delight at being able to tap into the shared intimacy that has endured creates a unique chemistry for rekindled romances. Many women I talked to have experienced variations on the same-guy/different-times theme. Donna Hanover—Rudolf Giuliani's unceremoniously dumped wife—has written a whole book about those love stories—including her own—called *My Boyfriend's Back*. When things click this time around, they cite the comfort of knowing each other—you can skip the first-date narrative (what a relief!)—combined with the mystery of not knowing what more there is.

Of course a lot can happen in those lost years, including big changes to the character that used to be there, and historic trust can be betrayed by unexpected cruelty. When a college boyfriend called fifty years after they dated, it seemed to Rochelle like "a fairy tale come true—Harvard man returns to Smith girl he'd rejected." She "plunged into a passionate love affair with a man who was married, but who insisted that his marriage was basically 'over.'" Two and a half years later, she says, "the passion had eroded. What had seemed a magical relationship had grown tawdry." He had no intention of playing out a fairy tale—or leaving his wife. Rochelle thought she knew her old boyfriend, but, it turns out, having shared those early chapters of their lives wasn't enough.

Many women find that the most dramatic change that has taken place over time is not in the old flame but in their perception of him. As our priorities change in the Second Adulthood shake-up, the kind of love we are looking for and attracted to is reordered. A "jerk" is now a thoughtful companion. A "dream boat" has become a bore. Some of the flashier traits that seemed so important then pale next to deeper virtues that have matured. At the same time, life experiences that have challenged the soul enrich the potential for loving compatibility. What the childhood sweethearts couldn't sustain then can become what sustains them now.

In Beth and Ned's love saga, all the stars shifted in the years between their tormented first romance and the second. Their long-ago first affair was intense and chaotic and very romantic. Ned, the brother of a classmate, was eight years older when they met, and an age discrepancy that big was a major differential. In those early years, the relationship was all intense conversations about life, literature, and justice, but not romantic. When Beth went off to college, they picked up where they left off and "talked and talked and talked." They would get together on school vacations. Finally, says Ned, with a loving glance at Beth, "I said I wanted to kiss you." Her reply is part of their thirty-year lore: "I have to go to the bathroom."

After three tumultuous years, they broke up. They simply

couldn't make it work; it was agonizing to be where they were, and they weren't emotionally or psychologically equipped to go anywhere else with the relationship. Both were devastated, and both married other people soon after. "I intentionally went for something different," says Ned, "for somebody who seemed stable and grounded and mature, to, you know, 'cure me' from my wild ways. I felt that all that passion had done for me was to make me unhappy, and make other people unhappy too." By the time he and Beth refound each other, he and his wife had grown apart and their daughter had just gone off to college, leaving the marriage even more empty.

Beth had been less thrown by the end of their affair; she married a musician "a lot like Ned," who had also been in a band when she knew him, and was quite happy. But when their children came along, she and her husband found themselves living in different time zones: night (he, the musician) and day (she, the primary parent). Although the breakup of the marriage was sad, the single years that followed became very empowering for Beth. She raised their two boys, built a career she loved, and went about her life with increasing happiness. "I didn't want my marriage to end. I really, really liked being married," she says. "But by the time Ned and I reconnected I really liked being alone. I mean, I *loved* having my house to myself." There were some things she missed, though—"sex occasionally, someone to travel with, and someone to call when you get home from a trip."

She is now forty-six; Ned is fifty-four. When they agreed to meet in the misty park where they first kissed (they have remained serious romantics), they had not seen each other for twenty-seven years. Beth had tried to stay in touch, but Ned rebuffed her efforts; the memories were still too painful. Once, she recalls, he actually said, "I don't know why you would call me. It's way in the past, and I have a life now; it's just a part of my adolescence." Finally, a few years later, after she called about a mutual friend who had died, they began e-mailing. They fell into easy correspondence about books and family, and Ned took note of some appealing changes. "There was a lot of talk about politics, and I was surprised because my memory was of someone who wasn't really interested in politics. And," he adds, "I had this great sense that you were this grown-up person. I wasn't older than you anymore." They have been living together for a year now and Ned's divorce is in process.

They spend a lot of time together, but, says Beth, giving as good a definition of *interdependence* as any I have heard, "we are both very autonomous people; I guess you'd say we have a shared autonomy." To reach that point, though, "we had to live our entire lives," she maintains. "We had a lot of growing up to do. If we had stayed together then, I don't think we'd be together now. This past weekend we were with some friends, and a man in his late fifties said, sort of offhandedly, 'There's no love like young love,' and I said, 'That's *so* not true.' I feel sorry for everybody who's eighteen, because they have to be in love as an eighteen-year-old instead of as a forty-six-year-old."

An emotional reunion with those who knew you then and love you now is unique; it creates a continuity between the past and the future that contributes to a sense of integrity—an interdependence—within the events of a lifetime. Reviewing those historic relationships also provides early clues to the authenticity we are seeking now. This New old Intimacy can truly help us grow up for real.

Chapter 7

Untangling Family Ties

> These are deep childhood attachments that through
> chance and tragedy were lost from view, but which, many
> decades later, memory may bring to light again. Recovery
> of and gratitude for these lost loves can be enormously
> healing.
>
> —George Vaillant, M.D., *Aging Well: Surprising*
> *Guideposts to a Happier Life*

There is one category of lifelong love (and hate and anger and loyalty and profound intimacy) that doesn't wait until everyone grows up. The hopelessly entangled relationships among family members that go back to the beginning of time offer fewer options for regrouping, and virtually no options for divorce. Yet as we make the transition to our

Second Adulthood, many of those bonds will be strained by the changes we are engaged in; indeed, we won't be able to move on unless we outgrow some of the patterns we have engraved on our lives, including behaviors that bind us to brothers and sisters, as well as parents.

Unlike childhood friends who bring the past into the present, family dynamics set up rivalries, barriers, and roles that define the past and overshadow the present. "I was the family clown," Carly Simon once said. "My sister was the mediator between me and my parents," another woman told me. Fran, who talked so passionately about her circle of childhood friends, has four sisters with whom she is very close, but, she observes, "in some ways the connection supersedes the relationship I have with my sisters. Because," she adds laughing, "with sisters it's not voluntary; you're stuck with each other. And you can't be as open about a lot of stuff."

Because we are "stuck with each other," no matter whether siblings are intimate friends or hardly see or think of one another, we operate on the assumption that the mode of coexistence we have worked out growing up is fixed. We are prepared for the annoying behavior or generous attention or cold distance or precious camaraderie we have come to expect from a brother or sister. We are probably not prepared for the intense reengagement required when, as so often happens to the "sandwich generation," an aging parent needs to be cared for at the same time that the siblings are deep into caring for their own families. It is rare that the grown children shift smoothly into an efficient caretaking team wherein each player's contribution is based on a reasonable evaluation of availability, personal expertise, and skills, finances, and geography. Instead, all those factors complicate the situation and activate lifelong resentments and control issues. "I live nearby and visit my mother every day," a man told me recently, "but when my brother shows up for an hour once every couple of months, he is the 'good son.'"

There are conflicts over money and over medical decisions. And new stepsiblings, stepspouses, and siblings-in-law bring their own baggage to the mix. As Mary Kay Blakely, whose large and loving family ultimately regrouped, writes in her forthcoming book, *Holy Days of Obligation: Becoming My Mother's Keeper,* "Mom's prolonged decline revealed family fault lines, shifted aortic attachments, and exposed secrets of gone civilization we grew up in." For Mary Kay—who is now sixty-two—the second act of caretaking hit just as she was emerging from the first and shifting her attention to her future. "My life started going in reverse ten years ago, shortly after my sons were finished with childhood and struck out on their own. My firstborn is now a father and my mother is increasingly becoming my child." She is on her own, but she is not just Mary Kay. She is, she realizes, also Daughter, Sister, Mother, and Grandmother. "It is a chore trying 'to thine own self be true' when there are four of you," she observes wryly. Every one of those roles will be rewritten as she and her siblings cope with their mother's dementia and MK struggles at the same time to stay in touch with herself and map out what's next for her.

OUR MOTHERS NOW

Even if we are not caring for our mothers, and even if we rarely spend time with them—even if they are no longer alive—the emotional status of our relationship with them is a major factor in our ongoing reinvention. The intimacy between a woman and the woman who gave birth to her has its own unique mix of physical, psychological, and gender forces within each of them. No matter how independent and grounded we have become in everyone else's eyes, in our own we are barely out of our teens in relation to her. Any attempt at resolution is a replay of the adolescent struggle to establish a strong and independent identity without stretching the bonds of love too far. Again, as we update the various realms of our love life, the challenge is to take the next step, whatever it is for each of us, from dependence to independence to interdependence. Especially with our mothers and especially now, establishing mutual freedom without neglect, acceptance without pity, devotion without guilt, is the way forward.

Making those adjustments is especially discomfiting for a generation that never resolved the tensions between the rewards and sacrifices of love and motherhood. Ambivalence is a consequence of the history we made, an ironic subtext to the narrative of our liberation. When we were young and outraged, our efforts to rectify historic injustices obscured the fact that those efforts put us in direct conflict with the very women whose abuse we thought we were avenging. In the course of exposing mistreatment of women, the phrase "blaming the victim" came to describe how rape victims, abused wives, and welfare mothers were victimized a second time by laws and attitudes that held them responsible for what happened to them. We didn't consider that our mothers were unjustly blamed victims too. Writing about us as we were in those unforgiving days, social psychologist Terri Apter observes, "Their mothers had, as they saw it then, bequeathed them a defective feminine nature. They had colluded with a society that restricted and even punished their efforts at self-correction."

Just think back to the wardrobe rebellions we undertook against the feminine establishment. If Mom wore a bra and girdle, we wore neither; if she wore skirts, we wore pants; if she wore high heels, we wore combat boots. In many ways, the more extreme among us modeled themselves on everything their mothers weren't, and most of us did so to some degree. Over the years, the adversarial model persisted. Whenever we reviewed our strained relationships with our mothers, it seemed necessary to assign blame. One of us had to be wrong, and it was usually her: "It's her fault that we weren't closer"; "I was right and she was wrong about how women 'should' behave"; "She abandoned me by going to work; she should have been a 'real' mother"; "She was just a housewife and didn't stand up for herself."

Now, though, we have mellowed in most ways, and the gray areas between *either* and *or* look more intriguing and much more true than they did; *both/and*—a less judgmental worldview—is now possible, and it offers much more room to maneuver. In dealing with our mothers, Apter writes, we are poised to create a balance "between this need to discover our female history through our mother, and the wish, which so many of us live with for so long, to free ourselves from her shadow." If we can replace "the impulse to complain about our inheritance with the need to understand it," we can find an accommodation with our mothers that is—at long last— liberating. The common ground is to be found in empathetic attention to her story, which we may not have tried to understand before. "In accepting her," Apter concludes, "we may be accepting our own femininity—which we can do when we feel strong enough to mold it to our own values and needs."

My friend Gretchen is that rare daughter who looks forward to time with her mother with the same delight and enthusiasm that she feels for her good friends, and when they are together, she and her mother talk about the kinds of things friends talk about. They share the stories of their lives on an ongoing basis. Such sharing can also make more room for tolerance. Essayist Natalie Angier is bound to her mother by the knowledge that she is the only person who will put up with Angier's politics. "I can say anything to my mother," she writes, "bitch and thunder and claptrap against all the world's misogynies and idiocies, and my mother won't recoil from me, or roll her eyes or belittle my complaints. Most of the time, she agrees with what I am saying, and when she doesn't we at least can fight loudly about the issue." Elsewhere, though, Angier admits, "I've gone through long stretches of hating my mother mindlessly and obsessively." "We daughters," she concludes, "like pit vipers, have nonretractable fangs."

As we daughters grow up again, though, the emotional truth of the relationship both then and now needs to be excavated from a lifetime of accumulated detritus. Sometimes the truth is not heartwarming. Nancy is an extreme, but not unusual, case. Her upcoming fiftieth birthday will mark the first anniversary of a liberating break with her toxic parents. Until then she had tried to thrive despite her father's contempt for the aspirations of girls and women and her mother's equally pernicious undermining of her efforts. ("She didn't want me to do better than her," Nancy believes.) Everything blew up, appropriately, in a cemetery where the family had gathered to unveil the gravestone of a relative. Since renouncing her parents, her career has taken off, she divorced her husband of eighteen years, and she realized that she is gay. For Nancy, making peace with her family meant giving up on making peace with them. Fifty will certainly be new for her.

Amy Ferris, who wrote *Marrying George Clooney: Confessions from a Midlife Crisis,* is in her midfifties; she has had a hard time too. While she was growing up, her mother was severely depressed and unavailable and, Amy suspects, never really happy about having children. Amy dropped out of high school, struck out on her own, and made a lot of choices that backfired. But she doesn't regret those decisions, she says, because "every fuckup, every bad move, every pain and suffering, got me to here," which is exactly where she wants to be.

The review of her own life was prompted by long hours contemplating her aged mother, who was by then bedridden and frequently violent and incoherent. Who *is* this woman? Amy wondered. She could no longer ask her mother directly, but sitting at her bedside day after day, she began to see "in her eyes in her face in her creases in her body that she has too many regrets and pains and wishes." When Amy lays her own life story alongside her mother's, she sees a stark contrast: While her mother's life seems thwarted in many ways, hers features "a strong, independent, emotional, by-the-seat-of-your-pants, impulsive, joyous, funny, willful, powerful, strident, passionate, talented, happily married, *and childless* woman." (She has never wanted to have children, Amy says).

She also makes a stunning connection with the mother who showed so little interest in her as a child. "I have become," she concludes with amazement, "the woman, the very woman, whom my mother had always wanted and wished to be." Ironically, that moment of empathy gave her a glimpse of the maternal approval—albeit darkened by regret and rendered in the negative—she had longed for. Small consolation, but enough to damp down some of the fires of resentment.

I too am contemplating my mother's story—and mine—as I sit by her bedside. Until she began to fail, I had convinced myself that I had "outgrown" her years ago. Our pattern of speaking across each other had settled into an almost conflict-free way of relating. I can't remember a time when I shared my dreams and doubts with her; she would make an effort to draw me out, but I felt so uncomfortable with the "femininity" she practiced that even in the years when we had marriage and children in common, I doubted we spoke the same language. I also kept my resentments and disappointments to myself, which is how we achieved such a peaceful coexistence. For her part, she marched defiantly to her own drummer. But now as she gets weaker, she seems more innocent, less defiant, and I have softened my defenses and begun to wonder about what *she* didn't tell *me*.

As it turned out, by the time I became curious about her life, she had forgotten most of it. But I was able to assemble some clues from my own memory. For example, it was my mother, never a great reader, who sent me a copy of Betty Friedan's *The Feminine Mystique* soon after it came out; I was surprised by the gift, but I didn't think to ask her why she found it such an important book to share with me. Was she trying to tell me what her life was like? Was it a call for help to rescue her from that life? Was she proselytizing for the current protest movement, "women's lib"—another of her political passions that began with "ban the bomb" marches and included animal rights and campaigning for countless candidates?

Ten years later, I was totally immersed in "women's lib" but it never occurred to me to consider my mother a woman in the process of liberation. I now see that widowhood set her free—at fifty—to embark on a perilous and very lonely quest for accomplishment. By sheer willpower, ambition, and intelligence she worked her way through college, graduate school, a career in social work—and a Ph.D. at eighty-two!

Throughout, she was still marching to a solitary drummer. She had almost no friends. Although she was ahead of her times in terms of independence, she was very much of her time—the forties and fifties—when it came to trusting other women. In her mind, everyone—including her own sisters—was a rival who envied her successes and would betray her if it served their purposes, especially if a man was involved. This was not a totally ill-founded suspicion, given the times and given that her beauty made her a target of envy. She went through life without experiencing that intimacy and trust in other women that I can't imagine being without. It is hard for me to picture what it was like having no one to share doubts and concerns with, especially about raising her children. She was on her own there too.

My heart goes out to that solitary and brave woman. Despite my carefully tended resentments and disappointments, I have come to see something more meaningful to me as her daughter than my (albeit justified) gripes—she did the best she could, which wasn't at all bad. In belated gratitude, I've been telling her that often and giving her long hugs. I know how much she needs that physical and emotional affirmation—because I need validation and reassurance from my children too. Every mother does.

This poignant revelation is evoked beautifully in Kate Walbert's novel *A Short History of Women*. It is the interwoven story of four generations of feisty but unfulfilled women. At the end, Dorothy, who is seventy-eight, takes to blogging, unbeknownst to her daughters. In her blog she describes herself this way: "I did what I was told to do, or rather, what I believed was required of me. . . . I was a housewife in the sixties and seventies, and though I had many friends, we'd rarely talk of more than our children and our husbands' jobs.

There were times in the middle of the night when I would wake and walk into my children's room. It's the one place where I felt whole, somehow, and I would often just sit on the edge of one of their beds, thinking." Recently though, she has divorced her husband of fifty years, been arrested for antiwar protests, and become obsessed with Florence Nightingale, whose courage, determination, and optimism she admires. Inspired by the World War I nurse's fortitude, "DT" is, she writes, "trying to find my OWN VOICE. I am trying to SAY WHAT I MEAN. I am BEING PRESENT."

One of her daughters, who has also divorced her husband and is living alone, happens upon the blog, identifies the author, and is, at first, horrified. Now in her early fifties, she is doing some soul-searching of her own. The more she thinks about her mother's outrageous act, the more she empathizes with her state of mind. Using the pseudonym Robinsnest, she writes back: "I find it is the dark of the night when you least expect it—whatever this thing is—regret, perhaps, but not, it is bigger than that, more epic, somehow, padded and full and weirdly historical: this restlessness, this discontent. Now it rises up to knock your breath out. Was this what you felt, DT, when you sat on the edge of our beds?" By tucking in the small word "our," Robinsnest is extending her hand across the abyss between herself and her mother. She goes on to address her contemporaries, women whom she has never met, but whom her generation has come to trust with the truth, "Is this the same feeling for any of you?"

ROLE MODELS OF OUR OWN

We have gone through so many transformations as we shed the roles we were raised to play, that looking into the uncharted future, we expect that there is still more to discover. About becoming who *we* want to be. We long for someone to show the way. Like Robinsnest, we look for a connection with our mothers' experience, but we are unlikely to find the guidance we need there; instead, like her, we look to the women alongside us in a common search for authenticity. An important source of the New Intimacy is there.

Although there are few role models for us, in the sense of mentors and mothers sharing their wisdom about coping with experiences they have been through, we are establishing a team of guides and protectors. They are us. It has not escaped me that when I call us "we," I am referring to women who are far enough apart in age—roughly forty-five to seventy-five—to be mothers and daughters, technically different generations. But when it comes to finding support, wisdom, and intimacy that will sustain us moving forward, we are a single generation. Together we struggled to stay afloat in the midst of earth-shattering changes for women in our first adulthood, and we are struggling to assimilate those changes in our Second. I call the women who are meeting the same challenges

Horizontal Role Models. They are part of this discussion about intimacy and motherhood, because they come from the same place we did—not necessarily the same town or the same college or the same family, but the same starting point. They are inventing this unprecedented stage of life alongside us.

Still, it is surprising that women coming from a span of decades can bond as equals. I was struck by this miraculous affinity in the course of moderating a discussion among twenty women; we talked intimately about everything from anger to sex to spirituality. After two hours I realized we had not yet brought up the last taboo. So I asked the women to go around the room and each tell her age. For the first time all afternoon the room fell silent. Eventually, though, everyone confessed; the range was from forty-eight to seventy-four, yet we had no problem laughing, understanding, sharing openly, totally on the same page. Our common bond is that whether we were adolescents or mothers at the time, we're all daughters of the 1970s and 1980s.

The events of our young adulthood shaped us as much as World War II shaped "the greatest generation." It wasn't a matter of individual political persuasion or activism or involvement in any of the many societal changes that took place. To be alive then was to be affected. To take just one example, one that is particularly close to my tomboy heart: Whether we are now forty-eight or seventy-four, we were around when, in 1972, a lawsuit (filed by a mother and daughter) opened Little League to girls and when, in 1973, Title IX opened college sports to women in parity to men. Some of the twenty women at that meeting were only in grade school back then. They got to high school in time to join the explosion of enthusiasm for girls' sports. For others of us it was too late to take the field, but we experienced empowerment through sisters, cousins, and, yes, daughters. As girls put on uniforms and formed soccer leagues, and college women took up track, they and we on the sidelines all learned about much more than sports. We learned about teamwork and trusting other women; we learned the pleasures of open competition instead of manipulative subterfuge. We learned about sweating and physical strength. We learned it was okay to go for it ourselves, rather than just cheer others on.

As our "generation" broke through job barriers, financial double standards, unfair laws, and restrictive social practices, we defined women in new terms. As we may not be able to do with our mothers, with Horizontal Role Models we can refer back to shared experiences and forward to shared discoveries. The more we explore our potential to grow, the more those witnesses to our beginnings have to contribute. And the more attention we pay to untangling the web of our primal love relationships and establishing the openness, generosity, and mutual respect of the New Intimacy, the better we can reweave the individual strands into a safety net going forward.

Chapter 8

A Second Chance at Getting It Right

Nobody can go back and start a new beginning, but
anyone can start today and make a new ending.

—Maria Robinson, *From Birth to One*

When *Zoomer* magazine, a Canadian publication for people
over fifty, asked its readers what they would do if they had to
live their lives over, the top five answers had to do with
choices they had made about love and intimacy: "I would
have had more children"; "I wouldn't have had children"; "I
wouldn't have married my first husband but still had the
same children"; "I would have never married young"; "I
wouldn't have settled for less." For most women in this
group, children are no longer an option, but in terms of their
deepest relationships, Second Adulthood can be a do-over.

A second chance at establishing the kind of intimacy, the kind of interdependence, that we weren't equipped for or weren't looking for the first time around.

Statistics predict that more than half of the American women over forty-five will be single—due to divorce, widowhood, or because it has always been that way. Many will not find—or rekindle—the love they wish for; others may not wish for romantic love at all, because they have been-there-done-that and have other sources of intimacy and support in their lives. But some will find what feels like the Real Thing—at last. And it is very likely that what they will find will be different from what they had been looking for when they were younger.

One of the strong drives in these years is to get to the heart of who we truly are and figure out how that person wants to experience her second chance at growing up. That inquiry involves reevaluating the choices we have made in our lives so far. With that self-knowledge, we recalibrate our priorities and our relationships, and we respond to choices that come before us now differently from how we did in the past. And the hopes and dreams we are uncovering bear little resemblance to those we have held for so long. That is why efforts to revive a long-standing wish list will feel unsatisfying. We draw fuel for these new beginnings in the very condition that is too often considered the denouement. "There is no greater power in the world than the zest of postmenopausal women," Margaret Mead said.

We are most definitely not who we were chemically. At menopause we experience a reallocation of the estrogen-progesterone-testosterone mix that, while it accounts for the "zest" Meade talks about, also accounts for those days when we are dazed and confused. The hormonal upheaval affects energy, sex drive, and assertiveness. Yet, interestingly, while the mood can be changed and the libido perked up chemically, no pill can replace the capacity of a respectful and supportive partner to get a woman going. In other words, no matter how hot or how "young" our chemistry is, the emotional context has to reflect where we are now.

Christiane Northrup, a leading authority on the menopause experience, confirms that a testosterone booster can produce "increase of libido, increased sexual response, increased frequency of sexual activity, increased sexual fantasies, and increased sensitivity of erogenous zones," but, she adds, real sexual awakening requires that "a woman's intimate relationship is healthy and mutual." The trust and openness that characterize the New Intimacy are prerequisites this time around, Northrup maintains, because, among other things, "at midlife . . . a woman is less likely to sweep resentment under the rug."

Such interrelated emotional, social, and physiological realignments make for a bumpy passage, and the winds don't blow out to sea overnight. The period of turmoil, self-doubt, and confusion—the Fertile Void—sounds like the last place we would want to be when we are poised for a second chance at love. But by experimenting with new ways of doing things and new and more authentic ways of interacting with those we want to love, we can begin to enjoy the possibilities within the confusion and experience the freedom of not knowing. In the process, we will reshuffle our requirements for intimacy and review the investments we are prepared to make. For those of us in long-term relationships, that means figuring out how—or if—the new wine fits into the old bottles. Those setting out again may surprise themselves by what—or whom—it is they want now.

THE GRASS IS GREEN, BUT IS IT GREENER?

With more options on the table, it is tempting to fantasize about all of them. During the ten years that the book club Katrina Kenison (author of *The Gift of an Ordinary Day*) belongs to has been meeting, "there have been two divorces and both women are dating again, involved with new men," she wrote me. "The conversation around this is always so interesting—those of us in long marriages envy the dates, the spontaneity, the romance, the independence, the second chances. We want to hear all the juicy details. And yet I know my dear friends also envy us in a way, for our old, solid unmysterious relationships," she says. "These two women, ages 61 and 50, both look fantastic," she goes on, "but then I realize they are working really hard to look so good, in a way that us solid-marrieds aren't, because we don't have to. The grass is always greener, I guess. But I can tell you this: the seven married women are definitely living vicariously through our two bold and beautiful friends who are out there risking all in new relationships."

As in the case of Katrina's friends, divorce is a clear marker on the way to what's next in the relationship department. The majority of single women over fifty are divorcées, and the majority of those divorces were initiated by women finally in a position to escape constant conflict, deficient affection, emotional or physical abuse, or simple emptiness (as in the case, we are told, of Tipper and Al Gore). Divorce is one of life's most wrenching experiences—financially as well as emotionally (research shows a 20 to 30 percent drop in standard of living for women and a 10 to 15 percent *gain* for men). Yet most women emerge more optimistic and happy with their lives than many of their married friends. They have found that breaking free of a bad marriage, like other traumatic Second Adulthood experiences, was empowering and prepared them for becoming themselves at last. "I'm in charge of my life now," Winfred told Ashton Applewhite, author of *Cutting Loose: Why Women Who End Their Marriages Do So Well,* "and I realize, 'I've done this. I've created this. This life.'" "Divorce has one good outcome," Martha told me. "It forces you to get to know yourself."

"People were very surprised when we got divorced," says

Jill of her decision to leave her first husband. Pert, warm, and full of enthusiasm, she felt "dead" in the marriage. "We weren't fighting all the time, he wasn't cheating; I wasn't cheating," she explains. "There was just a lack of real love, there was a lack of romance; there was a lack of sharing things other than our children." She tried to bring the marriage to life. "We went to three marriage counselors and three rabbis, and everyone said to me, 'Look, if you want to stay in this marriage, this man will never change, that's the way he is; you have to make that decision.' I went on a little further, but I started getting depressed; there was something inside of me that was very lonely and longing to communicate, to share things." So she told her bewildered husband that she needed to end the marriage. "I didn't want to break up my family—that was the hardest part; I cried over that, I really, really cried. I felt and still feel guilty about my children. And I really believe that my breast cancer a couple of years later was a result of that inner turmoil."

But Jill never regretted the decision. Many years later, she was happy being "an independent single woman" whose children were doing well, with a job she enjoyed and a series of "male friends." She had no interest in looking for love. But her kids pushed her to sign up on JDate, a Jewish online dating service. "I met some very nice people that weren't for me," she recalls. Then along came Charlie. "There was one line in his profile that really resonated for me, where he said, 'I would like to meet a woman who likes the finer things in life but knows how to give back to the community.'" She contacted him, and they arranged to meet at a restaurant. "He walked in and it was just like—boom! He looked at me; I looked at him. . . . I hadn't felt that way in I don't know how long, maybe from when I was a teenager. We were talking for an hour and a half before we ordered anything, and the waiter kept coming over, and we kept apologizing. We had the longest dinner possible, and later when he put his arm around me and I felt this electricity—there was real chemistry." The sex, which happened soon after that "magical" night, "was really very amazingly passionate. We have this wild chemistry going to this day!"

After that first date, Jill stayed up all night wrestling with a dilemma. "After he told me about the grief he had gone through with his wife, who he had lost from breast cancer, how was I going to tell him that I had a history of breast cancer?" She did tell him, the next day, and his reply was: "It doesn't matter. I just fell in love with you last night and that's it."

As the relationship developed, so did the real-life challenges of starting over when both partners bring extensive baggage with them. Who is going to move into whose community? How will the kids get along? What financial setup does each have in mind? And how will they adjust to each other's previous domestic experience? Charlie had been married for his whole adult life and, as Jill put it, "didn't have lots of dating experience. I did. And it was very painful for him to think about me with other men. 'But this is part of who I am,' I said." Upon reflection, though, she realized that who she is now is not who she had been, and while her past was part of her present, she didn't have to push it. "I realized that he's kind of an old-fashioned guy; it's hard for him to accept this, so I got rid of all my pictures of every boyfriend that I ever had."

Whether there are children at home to be factored into the equation or active parenting is in the past can make a major difference the second time around. While their children were the primary bond between Jill and her first husband, they were the gulf between Margery and Roy, who became totally engaged in his work when their children came along. "Roy and I met in college, and he was adorable, he was bright, we had a lot in common, we both loved reading, we both loved eating; he loved eating more than I did, because he turned out to be quite obese in the end. I loved cooking, he loved eating, and we started having children right away. Initially there was a great deal of enthusiasm and love and all that other stuff," she remembers. "Then we kind of went separate ways, with him devoting most of his energy toward his career and me devoting my energy around the children," one of whom had a chronic disease. He became irritable, withdrawn, and rejecting. Nevertheless, they stayed married for forty-two years and divorced only a few years ago.

"The children caused stress in the marriage," Margery recalled, "because he really wanted to be the only child, and so the more children we had the more stress we had as a couple; I was devoted to the kids, and he was jealous." The lonelier Margery got, the more she wanted another child—and the less Roy cared about whether or not they did. Despite all the failings, sex was good throughout the marriage, and she insisted to friends that she was happy, even when one of them told her, "I'm not going to go out with you and Roy anymore because he doesn't treat you nicely."

"I always envisioned myself as part of a couple," Margery admits. "I knew I could go on my own, but I like caring for somebody, so that really feels good to me. I cared for Roy, I 'took care' of him—in fact I went on every diet that he ever went on—I went on Weight Watchers with him, and then when he went to this spa where they promulgated veganism, I became a vegan. I thought, I could do this, that's not a big deal, I love vegetables, and I can figure this out, so we became vegans. So, yeah, I felt like I was supportive." Yeah, right. Self-sacrificing is more like it.

As it turned out, being "supportive" to the extent of altering her own diet to suit Roy's was toxic in more ways than one. "When I got sick many years later, I went to a doctor, part of whose protocol is putting people on different diets for their body type, and based on their heredity and genetic makeup," she recalls. "And he said to me, 'Being vegan is the worst diet for you; you need meat and potatoes, you need fat, you need all those things that everybody's told not to eat, that's what your body needs, and I think being a vegan really made your body more vulnerable.'"

Throughout the marriage Margery maintained projects of her own and social activities; eventually she became a very successful real estate agent and later she got a master's degree in psychology. She liked being her own woman; it was the absence of intimacy she minded. If she had a second chance it would be in a relationship that offered the same degree of independence—and the same amount of good sex—but had the kind of interdependence that she felt she was entitled to.

Flash forward to Stan. Five years into the relationship, "the sex is really good. . . . I adore him." Stan is an intense and engaged companion, although, like Roy, he is very involved in his life outside the relationship. In fact, Stan is a lot like Roy. "There's some of the same characteristics," Margery admits, "but it doesn't bother me as much as it did with Roy, because with Roy I was raising children and he was MIA. Now if Stan is working and doing his thing, I can do my thing; it doesn't really bother me when he's irritable; we call it 'irritable brains syndrome.'" And both men are short.

When Margery and I talked, Stan had just left for a three-month trip to Africa. "When I met him, he told me of this lifelong dream he had of taking a sabbatical between his work life and his retirement, and that this sabbatical would be something that he did by himself." Unlike Roy's emotional abandonment, Stan's mission of self-discovery did not leave her a single parent. She could focus on parenting herself for a change. Having recently moved to the same city as Stan, she "went on a campaign to meet other women. I would go out whether he was home or not; I thought: He wants his own life, and I am going to build my life." This time around, Margery is thriving on the New Intimacy; the experiences that she is having outside of it are enriching the relationship. It is as though she were starting over in a revised context (no children at home) and experiencing the kind of mutual empowerment that eluded her the first time out, with the good—and thin—version of the man she fell in love with all those years ago.

NEW WINE IN WELL-WORN BOTTLES

Long-term marriages go through a series of chapters, any one of which could be the last. When there are children, they invariably dominate one of the most tumultuous chapters, and when they move on and leave the parents on their own, the empty nest can reveal an empty marriage. But in most respects each marriage has its own narrative with its own crossroads. Medical problems, financial crises, work issues, sexual malaise—or the indefinable desire for change that strikes at midlife—can set things off. Each stress point is a chance to give up or change direction. Changing direction can be as arduous as turning an ocean liner around; after all, everything is at stake and everything is on the table, and any recalibration of the emotional, financial, or psychological equilibrium is risky. But if the partners do reach the last chapter on terms that feel empowering to both—and not as weary warriors—it can be the most fulfilling chapter of all.

Megan is at a major crossroads. She doesn't know which end is up in her marriage, and she is not sure she is grounded enough to find out. "We are both in the process of 'recalibration,' which is both freeing and frightening," she says. "Will our relationship change so much that it is unrecognizable? Will the end result be worth keeping?" Can she become "an autonomous human being within the partnership" that has intertwined her life with her husband's in ways that were comfortable for so many years but have come to feel confining? Whatever the outcome, there is no turning back. "I need change to occur; otherwise I—we—will be stuck in the same stultifying, suffocating rut." That rut has a particular pothole that echoes a painful theme in Megan's mother's life. "I may be light-years away from my mother's experience, but I can see her in me in that I allow my 'crumple buttons' to be pushed too easily by my partner."

Unlike Megan, Wendy and her husband do not need to change course so drastically. While they need to make adjustments to their marriage, they can build on a relationship that has grown with the events of their life together. She sees her marriage in terms of the chapters of family life, during each of which both she and her husband made accommodations to the circumstances—and also to each other. So when the household was back down to just the two of them, they had the accumulated goodwill and negotiating skills to reinvent their mode of interdependence. "I had my son a year and a half after we got married," she begins. "I also put my husband through school, and had my daughter at twenty-one. Then he put me through school. My thirties marriage found my love being more comfortable as we settled into the choices we had made. . . . A lot of times the love was there to brace us as we raised our kids. The forties love seemed the toughest, I think. This was when our children both went away to college and we were home by ourselves for the first time. Money pressures (dreaded college expenses) seemed to interfere with 'love.' The changing of my aging sags and bumps on my body affected how I responded to my husband. But my fifties love couldn't be better. We are rediscovering our marriage."

Margaret literally fell in love again with the same man she married forty years ago. She sees three chapters in those years—the children, the rough times, and the best time ever. The rough times—when they got so far from each other that they separated for a year—felt like the finale. Looking back, though, she understands that it was during that time—she was in her fifties and very much adrift in the Fertile Void—that they revitalized their marriage by confronting the truth about their needs, resentments, expectations, and disappointments. Gloria Steinem's observation about politics certainly applies to domestic politics over the long haul: "The truth will set you free—but first it will piss you off!"

It wasn't a pretty picture back then, but today Margaret and her husband are relishing their second chance. When they got back together it was on terms that gave each of them more room to pursue their separate interests, more attention to and respect for each other's work, and more delight in who they were together. Their professional life, family life, and sex life are all thriving, and they are more in sync than ever before.

I can identify three periods of closeness and distance in my marriage too—being a couple, being parents, being ourselves. People often ask me about such a long marriage, and I tell them—and it's true—the first thirty-seven years were the hardest. During phase one we operated in a fairly traditional way, even though we were a two-career couple. When we got married, I was working at *Mademoiselle* magazine, where, back then, an editor's greatest accomplishment was not to work with the best authors but to add "his" name onto "hers" on the masthead. During the same time, Bob went from lawyering rather uncomfortably at an advertising agency to lawyering somewhat more comfortably at a law firm. Ultimately, in the early seventies, I went on to *Ms.* magazine, and he created his own firm, where he established the kind of nourishing community I was also becoming immersed in at *Ms.*

Outside the office, though, we socialized as a couple and did most things together. Generally he made the plans—where to travel, what movies to see—partly because he was very clear about what he wanted to do and partly because I was not clear at all. Back then, I simply couldn't access my preferences; I was more tuned in to what the others around me wanted. We walked like a couple, we talked like a couple, but we were not truly interdependent. Luckily for me, his ideas of what to do included things that were a lot of fun, and we really enjoyed each other's company.

We didn't have our children until we were entering our forties, more than fifteen years into our marriage, and parenthood brought the differences we had to the fore. Although we both adored our children, we disagreed about most child-rearing decisions, and especially about how much our lives should revolve around them. We walked less and less like a couple and talked less and less like a compatible one.

I often think of Hillary Clinton, who looked back on the trying times in her marriage and explained her decision to stick it out with the observation that she and Bill had "started a conversation" in 1971, and it was still going on. I think I was saying much the same thing when I looked over the rocky terrain and reminded myself, "At least I am never bored." The conversation changed big-time in the third chapter of our marriage.

It was only after we looked up from parenting, and I had come a long way toward finding my own voice—thanks in large part to the support and encouragement of the women's movement—that we could begin what felt like an authentic conversation, rife with opinions, unresolved disagreements, delightfully discovered *both/and* outcomes, honest criticism. Learning to say no and yes with conviction enabled me to hold my own in emotional and practical negotiations with him; in the face of honest blowback, he was more inclined to reconsider his *no*s. We were beginning to define ourselves as individuals within the marriage, making plans on our own, making mutually approved decisions, fighting as equals. It was enormously refreshing.

I don't know how much of the change in our marriage is due to my reinvented communication skills, how much to adjustments he made in response to what I had to say, and how much was part of his own mellowing and growing faith in the relationship. Our deepening intimacy expressed itself in quirky ways. For example, a very important new bond developed over our cats. While I was finding my inner assertiveness, Bob was finding his inner cat lover. Although he was not aware of it, he was also making a connection with me on a very intimate level.

I have had a cat at every stage of my life—Archie consoled

me as an adolescent; Roo kept me company as a lonely young woman in a strange city; Narouz was a soul mate, pure and simple; Olmo and Heathcliffe sat with me at dawn as I gathered my faculties to get the kids going, and *their* first cats, Sassy and Phyber, marked a new generation. Bob barely tolerated our cats—and my profound connection to them.

Then a few years ago we took in a twenty-year-old tough feline broad. I didn't adore her, but that may have left room for Bob to succumb to her gruff appeal. After she settled in, I would hear him "talking" to her, looking for her, pointing out her virtues and personality quirks—all the things we cat lovers do. By the time Winnie died, he had been hooked; I couldn't believe it when he observed one day how empty the house seemed. We have recently taken in my daughter's cat, and Bob is totally into Tito's charms. To a nonbeliever, a belated cat connection coming to life between husband and wife may not sound like a major step toward intimacy, but to me it is huge. I perceive his delight in the cats as a demonstration of an untapped well of tenderness that has extended through our shared enjoyment of Winnie and Tito—to me.

PICKING UP THE PIECES

Bob and I have the luxury of growing closer as we grow up this time around. A second chance that is the result of tragic circumstances certainly doesn't feel like a growth opportunity. There is nothing more debilitating than losing a life partner, and the prospects for putting your life back together look grim. After a time, though, when the grief begins to let up, a widow has to ask herself the same relationship questions that each of us is grappling with in our various situations: In the next chapter of my life, do I want more of what I had? Or something and someone totally different? Or do I want to go it alone? And how do I get moving?

For a widow in particular, the process of getting unstuck from the past can be a daunting prospect. Sara, who had lived a roller coaster of emotional and health issues with her husband, Bill, had also worked with him over the final ten years of his life. Together they ran a consulting business that benefited from her accounting background and his people skills. After Bill died, she decided to carry on without him. The hardest part, she discovered, was "stepping out of the background—being the person who called the shots." She had had some ideas of her own all along, but she was "really scared." It was months before she felt entitled to implement them. Today, she is still grieving over Bill, but the business is thriving and she can see a road ahead.

When I wrote about Joan and Robert B. Parker, the mystery writer, in *Inventing the Rest of Our Lives* it was because of their ingenious adjustment to marriage. Well into their long relationship they both felt burdened by the demands of living together and thought the marriage was over. But after living apart for a while, they found they missed each other's company. So they came up with a very creative solution: interdependent real estate. They divided their Victorian house into two apartments. Joan had a separate entrance to her second-floor rooms and Bob had the downstairs, including the kitchen, because he was the cook in the family. The setup gave them the freedom to come and go as they chose but still come home to each other. They lived happily that way for almost a decade until Bob died in 2010. They had been married for fifty-three years.

Joan was devastated, and the artifacts of their life together depressed her. Now that the whole house belonged to her, she realized that she had to make it hers. If redesigning their living quarters a decade ago had saved their marriage, then maybe moving the furniture around would help her cope now. She didn't replace Bob's things, but she moved some of them into less-used rooms and rearranged chairs and bookcases in others. The accumulated minor adjustments gave her a second chance at experiencing her surroundings and her daily life without eliminating Robert's presence. "I am not in this house of death, where such a sad thing happened, but a whole new house, a whole new landscape," she says now.

Of course the breakthrough, as Joan understands, was not about furniture but about mastery over the situation. "I was powerless to prevail over the turmoil, fear, grief, and uncertainty following Bob's sudden death," she says. On the other hand, she finds some control over "the inanimate objects inside my house. So I move, lift, reuse, re-recycle, drag, discover things, and in so doing actively transform my physical living space. And hope to Christ it empowers me to transform my emotional living space."

Only recently, after three marriages—one ended in divorce, the other two in widowhood—has Cassandra felt that she has the right to stake out an "emotional living space" of her own, and she intends to make the most of her second chance to inhabit it. She started out living in a commune in California, where she met and married a jazz musician. They hoped to have children, but although that didn't happen, they were happy for ten years. When he developed terminal cancer, she took care of him; the burden was lightened as much as it could be by the coordinated and wide-ranging support from the community they lived in. When she was forty-eight, she left the commune and moved to the other end of the earth— New York City. That is where she met her second husband, a high-powered, gregarious, and very rich man. "It was a *totally* different life" is her understated comment.

When husband number two developed heart problems, Cassandra took on the role of caretaker again, only this time there was no commune to back her up. She was on her own in a city she barely knew and far from the friends she needed. After he died, she was totally depleted and took off for New Mexico to regroup. Then, just as she stepped off the plane, *she* had a massive heart attack. Her body was screaming,

Wake up! "There was minimal damage to my heart," she says, "but my life completely changed."

The next two years were her Fertile Void. Financially secure for the first time, she lived by herself and concentrated on designing and building the house of her dreams. In the course of literally constructing a new life, Cassandra began to learn a thing or two about how she was put together. As so often happens, a significant revelation came from her body. "I went to an optometrist and he said, 'You know, you don't have any peripheral vision.' I realized that in order to survive I had developed tunnel vision. I only focused on what was in front of me." Her fixation was on men. "It has taken me ten years," she says of her withdrawal period, "to get a sense of who I am and what is important for me to function."

Cassandra recently met a widower, but she's not fixating on the relationship. "It remains to be seen what's going to happen here," she says, but whatever does happen, it will not be more of the same. For one thing, he is "a very different type" for her; "he looks at you when he talks; he asks questions, and he listens." More important, she is different too. She is more pragmatic about the prospect of another till-death-do-us-part relationship. "I worry about getting involved with another older man," she says. "What I am looking for at this point in my life is somebody to travel with and have fun with. What I want is a sense of joy and peace and doing some things that are worthwhile and being important to people and not trying to be somebody that somebody else thinks I should be."

CAN WE TALK?

Two qualities mentioned most often in second-chance relationships that weren't there before are good conversation—straight talk (*and* attentive listening)—and peaceful companionship—as opposed to past relationships many women described as "roller-coaster rides." Open communication and the mellowness that the years bring—not sweating the small stuff—are the bedrock of the New Intimacy in relationships that are being built—or rebuilt—to be shared.

Robyn hadn't found that kind of communion and maybe never would, but she wasn't about to commit herself to anything less. Which didn't mean in any way that she gave up on fun. For seventeen years after her second divorce, she dated widely and enthusiastically. "I was the happiest single lady around—and I had no desire to change that. None! Husband number two cured me of the whole marriage thing," she told me. "I dated a lot. And mostly the men who asked me out were younger, sometimes a whole lot younger. It was fun, but I didn't find anyone that I wanted to spend even a weekend with, much less live with full-time. I didn't want to raise a man, just date him; and I need to be able to talk with him as well."

Then a caring man with whom she could really talk entered her life. "I ran into a man that I had known, but never dated, in high school. He came to the bank where I worked at the time; we chatted; he left. Over the next six months or so he would come in every now and then; we'd talk, and then he would leave," she recalls. They literally talked their way into each other's lives. "Just before Thanksgiving he called to make sure that I would not be spending the holiday alone. From Thanksgiving until Christmas we talked on the phone at night and wrote letters back and forth. Christmas night he came by the house to show me the print that he had been working on while we were chatting. I could have told you that night that he would be a permanent part of my life. It just felt right! We married a year and a half later—there were no qualms, no fears, no hesitation, just pure joy!"

Joy means something very different to Robyn this time around; the peaceful companionship is a new and precious ingredient. "It's a quieter kind of thing than you feel in your twenties," she says, "but it is so much nicer. There isn't all that pain and angst that you have when you are younger. I still get a little shiver when my husband walks into the room. He just makes me feel good—special. We have such fun together—we spend a lot of our time just laughing over nothing."

REORIENTING SEXUALITY

For some women, who have been heterosexual until now, the joy of midlife love turns out to be found with a same-sex partner. Sociologist Pepper Schwartz, who has been writing about sexuality for more than thirty years, has observed that "a lot of midlife women feel that they are more simpatico with women, and maybe this is the point at which they finally complete the picture. They feel that women are better listeners, more sympathetic, share better—play well with others—that they like those qualities in women. They have liked sex with men, but the relationships were not as fulfilling as women's friendships were. In that situation they may then say, 'well, what the hell. . . . yeah!'"

Grace and Amelia, whose egalitarian relationship I used as an example of interdependence, were close friends for years—until lightning struck Amelia at a Holly Near concert. Near "started singing the words, something like, 'Why does my love make you uncomfortable? It's love, only love, my love for a woman.' And all of a sudden my whole body responded. . . . I felt a physical attraction for Grace that was something more than for a close friend," she remembers. Grace felt the same way. About their second-act love, she says, "I sometimes think of the anthropologist Margaret Mead, who had three committed relationships. Her first was for children, her second was for intellectual exchange, and her third was for love. That third relationship was with a woman."

Coryn and Sally had also been friends before they became lovers. Neither had been with a woman before, but "at a certain point we both realized that we both would rather spend time with each other than anyone else," Coryn recalls. They got married in California, where they live, and when I talked to Coryn, who is forty-six, she was ecstatic; she had just found out that "we're expecting." Sally, who is ten years younger than Coryn, is carrying the pregnancy. Both had been married before, and Coryn has two teenage boys who live with them. As they had been friends for years, the boys knew Sally well, so when Coryn left the marriage, one son reassured her, "It would be a lot weirder if you were bringing home a strange man."

The sex was like "having a physical relationship for the first time," Coryn says. "I realized what fireworks are. I'd always heard that phrase but never understood it, and never experienced it before. That was really the turning point for both of us; we realized, 'Oh, my gosh, this is it!'"

The most unexpected testimonial to the joys of a woman connecting with her authentic self—sexual and otherwise—in a second-chance relationship comes from the former husband of a woman who "left him for another woman." Barbara had some lesbian relationships before their marriage, she told Paul at the time, but she was sure that was all over. Things went well until their twins were born. "After our kids were born and over the two years before the breakup, she wasn't the same woman that I had married, and she wasn't the kind of mother I thought she would be," Paul says. "But the minute she came out, and I was supportive of her, she almost instantaneously became happier and a better mother."

BEING LOVED

"Coming out," as Barbara did, is an apt metaphor for the true needs, desires, and passions—the loving—that can be set free in Second Adulthood. "Taking in," as in learning to accept and bask in undisguised devotion, is another monumental new experience for many of us. A big difference between love then and now is that now it is as much about being loved as about loving. The affirmation that comes from feeling entitled to be loved and respected is ground zero for the New Intimacy—regardless of the nature or duration of the relationship.

That is a total reversal of the catch-me-if-you-can style of courtship we spent our youth training for. In that scenario, a woman's self-esteem hinged on how well she hunted. If her prey gave up without a fight, he couldn't be worth the chase. A "nice guy" had to be some kind of jerk for being nice—to her. I can remember many conversations early on with bewildered friends who couldn't understand why they just weren't turned on to some otherwise appealing guy who praised and accommodated them. "Just too nice" was the kiss of death. We needed years of accomplishment, and, yes, independence before we accumulated what it takes to accept the prospect of—yes again—interdependence. "Those who have trouble receiving," Christiane Northrup observes, "attract those who have trouble giving."

Fran, who is divorced and not in a relationship, is stunned

by the choices her high-powered friends are making these days. "Many of my women friends who are going around a second time married men who—I don't want to say 'put them on a pedestal,' because that sounds too 1957, but men who are appreciators of women in a way that their first husbands were not—men who admire their spouses. They definitely treat them like, 'Aren't I lucky to have gotten her?' I know three people that this happened to—and in every case the woman had been married to kind of fast, sharp, very cutting kind of guys—they were all very successful; when they married again, they married guys slightly less successful but who treated them better. In every case that woman went, 'This is what I want—this is what I want.'" Fran was so sure that one match was doomed, she admits, that she "told her, 'Don't marry him.' I said, 'Don't go, don't.' I thought it would be a disaster. I liked the guy, but I thought she'd kill him, she'd roll right over him. It's turned out to be a very happy marriage. I was totally wrong." Fran hadn't accounted for the rising currency of the niceness factor.

"I would never have picked a man like this before, way too nice," Abigail told me. After her divorce she didn't date for fifteen years while her son was growing up. "I felt it was my duty to dedicate myself to my child," she explains. By the time her son turned eighteen, she was fifty and assumed "the fun was done." Then she met a man who is the "best, kind, thoughtful, generous to a fault, helpful, caring, et cetera, et cetera." He is also younger. "I am fifty-one and he is thirty-one," she added. "I never went looking for a younger man, never even thought about it, but, boy, is it awesome!" She isn't counting on happily ever after in the future, but "from where I'm sitting at this moment, it looks great."

WHAT'S DIFFERENT ABOUT YOUNGER MEN?

Women like Abigail represent another departure from the huntress model of meeting and mating. Instead of looking to tie a great "catch" into the big bow of marriage, they are reveling in low-maintenance fun. Many younger men are on the same wavelength, and find themselves attracted to experienced women. "Cougar in New York" was bewildered by the attention. In a letter to Dear Abby, she described her situation. "I am a fifty-nine-year-old woman who has been dating younger men in their forties. At first I refused, because I thought they were too young for me and people might laugh. Since then I have decided that as long as they know from the beginning that I'm not looking for a serious committed relationship, I'd be happy to go out. I have made some great friends and had some great times." Why, she wondered, were these young men attracted to her? "If I were to hazard a guess," Abby replied, "I'd say it's because many older women are independent, self-confident, worldly, and not looking for commitment."

Nicole Prouix-King and Sandra Caron, a therapist and a

professor of family relations, are studying age-gap relation-ships. They have found that younger men appreciate the maturity of older women, whereas older men are uncomfort-able dating strong women. For their part, the women don't need to bask in the reflected status of a partner; they are totally comfortable with a less-achieving man and no strings.

If many women have given up on "Mr. Right," the imagi-nary guy worth competing for, does that mean they are "set-tling" for second best? Not as far as I can tell, but there are still some who mourn his loss. Writer Lori Gottlieb speaks for them in her book *Marry Him: The Case for Settling for Mr. Good Enough*. Having never found Mr. Right, she now regrets all the "Mr. Good Enough"s she rejected along the way. She is contemplating a second chance. But when it comes to reconsidering Mr. Good Enough, "the bar is lower," she argues. "You may be more satisfied simply because you go in with fewer expectations, and then you're pleasantly surprised when you develop a stronger bond with the person than you had anticipated. I think the people who go in with these very high expectations about what kind of fulfillment they're going to get from the marriage and the partner are kind of set up for disappointment." What that analysis misses is the humble truth that Mr. Right was always someone else's standard; now we still have high expectations, but they are based on our own true needs. And a second chance is the opportunity to fulfill them.

I could go on endlessly with variations on the theme of second-chance love, but the point is just that—the variations are endless. Second Adulthood is about revising, reenergizing, and rediscovering intimacy in our lives and finding it in places we hadn't looked before. With each relationship we have the opportunity to replace one-upmanship with interdependence, emotional death with "zest" for living, and control with kindness.

Chapter 9

Care Getting—the Next Frontier

From the mountain tops of Judea long ago, a heavenly
voice bade his disciples, "Bear ye one another's
burdens"; but humanity has not yet risen to that point
of self-sacrifice; and if ever so willing, how few the
burdens are that one soul can bear for another!

—Elizabeth Cady Stanton, "The Solitude of Self" (1892)

The interaction between the caretaker and the cared-for is a
form of intimacy that life has familiarized us with in many
ways. The bond we form when we take responsibility for the
well-being of someone else is another of the relationships
that will be tested as we move forward. In terms of the New
Intimacy, though, that relationship is different from the others, because no matter how much love and goodwill there is

on both sides, power and responsibility lie in the hands of the caregiver and cannot be shared equitably with the care getter. Where the challenge lies—and where the New Intimacy is generated—is in the understanding between the caregiver's own self and her caregiving self.

Caretaking is still considered women's work—with men and society sometimes offering a helping hand. The failure of efforts to change that dynamic is one of the disappointments of our generation's social revolution. Child care is not yet a recognized societal responsibility, and women are still expected to be the more flexible parent, the one who rearranges her day, and her life, to respond to family demands. At the other end of the life cycle, aging parents evoke the same expectations. When, for example, a family gathers to discuss the care of a failing parent, the most likely person nominated will usually be female (especially if she is unmarried), regardless of any personal and professional commitments she may have. Statistics show that the chances of being cared for at home rather than being sent to a nursing home improve significantly simply if the one in need of care has two or more daughters or daughters-in-law.

Our other options have changed dramatically, but when it comes to caring for those we love, it seems that we are still forced to make a choice that Carol Gilligan described in her studies of adolescent girls between "having a voice and having relationships." Can we learn to speak up for ourselves when confronted with caregiving demands and responsibilities—many of which we may actually want to fulfill? Conversely, can we give the care that is needed without stifling the voice that speaks up for our own needs? And is there any way to minimize the guilt that attends the answer to either question? The New Intimacy is about learning to accommodate the impulse to care for those we love with the imperative of self-preservation.

Coping with that caregiving paradox is even more fraught at this stage in our lives, because we are attempting to reclaim some of our caring resources—to "do unto ourselves as we have been doing unto others." We are reining in the impulse to fix every misfortune, console every hurt, and support every wish at whatever cost to ourselves. As one woman put it, we "are going out of the emotional management business." In order to not give away more of ourselves than we can afford to, we need to develop some important criteria for give-and-take—interdependence—within even the most unequal caregiving relationship. When, we must discern, is a "need" a demand? When is loving care another name for boundless self-sacrifice? And how do you introduce "care *getting*"—the notion that caring for oneself has to be a primary component of any caring relationship—into the equation?

When you are in the midst of the situation, it may feel as though attending to your own needs requires more energy than you have left over from caring for someone else. But care getting is as essential for survival as the oxygen mask we are ordered to put on before attending to a child in an airplane emergency. Attending to loved ones, even vulnerable loved ones, cannot do them much good if you don't have the wherewithal to stay the course. Holding on to—or, heaven forbid, *asking* for—emotional oxygen for yourself is just as essential to the caregiving relationship. That is how the New Intimacy is established, even when one person is otherwise dependent on the other.

Once again the magic word is *no*. It is hard to say no to the needs of those we love, even if they are basically "wants." Especially when health issues are involved. But we are toughening up as we retrieve the self-affirming voice we lost in adolescence. Annie has discovered that this is an ongoing exercise for women of our generation. "I feel that I learned how to say no to people and demands during my husband's prolonged illness and death. I also learned how to ask for help and accept it gratefully. But as I've gotten older—I'm sixty now—it's been interesting to start seeing how older women are automatically assumed to be available, not only in terms of time but also in terms of being sort of a Giving Tree to everyone who wants an ear, a support, a cheerleader. As a teacher, parent, colleague, friend, I'm frequently surprised by how people, even ones who have known me for years, seem to think I've given up my own goals, preferences, and private time to participate in their events or activities."

Valerie is an extreme example of how caregiving can completely overrun any possibility of care getting. As a teenager her "parents placed a great deal of responsibility on me with my younger siblings," she explains. "I gave my all, even to the point of raising my youngest sister's two children after I was fifty years old." Like Annie, she became a Giving Tree. "When times were good for me, I shared my meager wealth or experience. When times were tough, I helped in any way I could." But then came the rude awakening. "When times were tough for *me*, it was not reciprocated. When an illness hit me hard, I lost my business, and the children I was raising hurt me terribly. I'd had enough!"

It was now or never. "I found my voice. I spoke my piece and told them it was time for me to think of myself and what was best for my husband and me.... The emotional bank is depleted. I think I surprised the hell out of the family." It was painful to renounce the boundless demands she had accepted, but she is determined to move on. "I made a promise to my mother before she died at a young age from cancer. Well, Mom, I tried. But when a ship is sinking there's a time to jump off. We're still a family; we still fight; but I'm not struggling to hold it together. We either sink or swim. Love me or leave me alone. *¡Basta!*"

JUST WHEN YOU THOUGHT THE COAST WAS CLEAR

With kids finally leaving home, a vision of the years ahead beginning to come into focus, and our relationships narrowing down to a precious chosen few, we are just beginning to explore what it means to care for ourselves—when the call comes. Parents who had been taking care of each other suddenly lose it; partners who had been mighty oaks crack; friends who had been there for you suddenly need your support; kids in crisis show up on the doorstep.

Ours is called "the sandwich generation" because we often find ourselves squeezed by responsibilities for children and for long-lived parents at the same time. When the responsibility is financial, the distinction between "needs" and "wants" becomes especially difficult to ascertain. The *AARP Bulletin* reported in December 2010 that 70 percent of its members still provide financial support for their grown kids and 40 percent are helping to support both kids and parents. The same AARP report offers the prospect of another dependent—ourselves. "The number of 75-plus households headed by single women is projected to grow from fewer than 6 million in 2010 to 13 million by 2050." We say that we don't want to be a burden on our children and also that we want to live out our lives as independently as possible. It will take more than wishing to make it so. Planning just may. We cannot lose sight of this practical side of care getting.

"You can't give up your life," well-meaning advisers remind you. But you will have to give up some of what your life was before the fateful phone call or event; the challenge of care getting is to hold on to enough of the rest.

Amanda is struggling to do just that. She is caring for her

husband of twenty years, whose physical ailments, as severe as they are, are more manageable than his chronic depression. "I live with someone who suffers from depression. That's the accepted term, I believe—rather than 'someone who is depressed,'" she explains. "But the odd thing about it is that he doesn't seem to suffer all that much. I, on the other hand, suffer a lot." Ethan has no energy to go anywhere, do anything, even take his medications; he is "unremittingly" pessimistic, critical, and bellicose; he has quite simply "lost all capacity for joy," Amanda laments.

His conditions and his medications combine to make him almost inert. "He is the slowest person anywhere," she says. "When I try to actually match his pace, it's like Marcel Marceau miming walking." At one point Amanda became so frustrated that she threatened to leave him if he didn't cooperate more. "I won't leave him," she admits. "I love him. But it's also true that I can't live like this."

There, in three phrases, is the plaintive cry of the desperate caregiver.

What makes their plight all the more cruel is that the so-called social support system seems fiendishly deaf to their cries. "It is hard to know where to turn for help," Amanda says. Besides the endless paperwork, battles with the insurance company, and managing a lengthening record of tests and consultations, those in charge of Ethan's case are unresponsive. "The psychopharmacologist has not returned our phone calls. The primary care doctor has always been busy, distracted, overbooked." Amanda has given up on the therapist too, "because Ethan never could follow through on anything we agreed on, and it was back to me, trying to figure out a way to make someone do things that would help him— except that the very thing that made them necessary was also making them impossible."

Amanda's advice to others in her situation: "Get out of the house, spend some time with yourself, rediscover who you are and what you like to do when you're neither cheerleading nor nursing." A seventy-three-year old writer named Elaine Long exemplifies the resourcefulness it takes to put Amanda's good advice into practice under the most debilitating circumstances. In a letter to *The Authors Guild Bulletin,* she reassures a woman who is worried that she is too old to get published by recounting her own story. Long didn't get her first book published until she was fifty-two; her second, at fifty-six. Then, just as she was getting under way as a writer, she had to shift gears and become "a double caregiver"—to her husband and her mother. Fifteen years later, four days after her seventy-third birthday, a CD of her songs was released. About that "lost" time, she writes: "Every one of the songs in *Lone Wolf Suite* rose in my mind as I drove the 64-mile round trip to the Alzheimer's unit where my mother lived, and my upcoming nonfiction book for caregivers is based on those 15 years of caregiving."

When my turn came, I was very lucky. My mother brought

a lot to the caregiving situation; she was basically healthy (it was her mind that was wandering), she was in remarkably good spirits, and she owned her own house. With the funds from a reverse mortgage (which allows a homeowner to draw upon the equity in the house during her lifetime), I was able to set up what my husband called "a one-woman nursing home." Although emotionally I had entered a parallel universe of anxiety and guilt, most of the components of my own life remained unchanged. At the beginning, she seemed to be managing on her own, and the demands on my time had to do mainly with logistics. I'd make her appointments (doctors, piano lessons, hairdressers, lunch dates), and take her there, though she kept offering to drive. Once she had literally forgotten about driving, I could bring in a "companion" a couple of afternoons a week to take her where she needed to go; on days when she had a doctor's appointment, I would build my time around meeting them there.

Besides scheduling and occasionally chauffeuring, I was also in charge of pill taking. At first all I had to do was remember to call twice a day to remind her to take them. As things progressed, I would have to wait on the phone until she took her pills to make sure she didn't leave them on the bedside table. Ultimately, someone—a "caregiver"—had to be there to give her the pills and make sure she ate regularly.

By then, the ring of my cell phone had become a heart-stopping siren. Someone hadn't shown up. She wouldn't take her pills. There was a leak in the attic. The heat went out. The caretakers ranting about one another. She fainted; should they call 911? They needed more cat food. Was it one of the doctors calling me back? Or was it what I came to think of as "the call"? I always felt one step behind the increasing care that she needed, but at the end (yes, during the time I have been writing this book she died) I got a glimpse of the kind of support that was possible if there was the political will to make it so. A home hospice team, consisting of a nurse, a doctor, a social worker, and a twenty-four-hour nursing hotline (all covered by Medicare), took charge of her care. After four years of anxiously managing her changing needs and crises as best I could on my own, I was finally able to concentrate on being with her. It was a gift.

Throughout, I was never in the position of having to sacrifice my own life for her care. Many much less fortunate women are trapped in situations that don't allow for even an hour off duty. Others are trying to do it all, caregiving while holding down a paid job. For the most part they are on their own. A recent *AARP* magazine's "Caregivers' Wish List" reported on the needs of the 65.7 million working Americans who are also caring for a family member. Their wishes are pitifully simple and outrageously neglected: a paid leave of absence from work—either hours in the week or a few weeks—to deal with a crisis; a tax credit or a government voucher program that pays minimum wage to the full-time caregiver, who has to forfeit her own salary; respite care—a qualified replacement available to take over while the caregiver takes a breather; transportation to and from medical appointments; knowledgeable guidance in discovering, accessing, negotiating, and navigating among needed services.

Mobilizing political pressure to enact responsible social policies can call attention to such needs, but change won't come soon enough for today's caregivers. So mobilizing your own circle of caring volunteers is an immediate necessity. Many times they want to help but don't know how. It is helpful to be specific in your requests—"Can you bring a supply of soup this weekend?"; "Can you help me with my taxes?"; "Can you research the visiting nurse options?"—and to extend each request to the person most likely to be able to carry it out; the "caregivers' wish list" is a good starting point.

CARE NEEDING

As hard as it is to rally a support team to help you care for someone else, it is even harder to ask for assistance when, sooner or later, you need help caring for yourself. By the time you are in your Second Adulthood, you probably have already had a medical crisis or are likely to have one. Heart disease is the primary cause of death among women over fifty, and the incidence rises precipitously after menopause. Cancer is the next biggest killer. Two or three out of one hundred women who are now fifty and up to four out of one hundred women over sixty will get breast cancer in the next ten years. HIV/AIDS is—but needn't be—a significant presence in our age group. Too many women think that if they can't get pregnant they don't need to use condoms, or are too new to the game to be comfortable insisting on using one. And Alzheimer's lurks behind every birthday.

However extensive the treatment, we want to manage our care and maintain our independence as best we can. In fact, a take-charge attitude can be part of the cure. Dr. George Vaillant, who researched the major longitudinal studies of adult development for his book *Aging Well,* found that "Objective good physical health was less important to successful aging than subjective good health. By this I mean that it is all right to be ill as long as you do not feel sick."

Charlotte had no intention of becoming sick when she fell ill. She is seventy-three, has never been married, and is fiercely independent; she was determined to be proactive about taking care of herself when she was diagnosed with thyroid cancer. She managed to cope with the surgery on her own, but was stymied when, due to a rare side effect of the operation—paralyzed vocal cords—she lost her voice. "In addition to not being able to speak," she says, "I had no energy. It was terrifying." And she had no interest in food. "I couldn't have any salt. They talked about putting a tube in my throat." Her friends and neighbors rallied to help her recover at home. One, a gourmet cook, put a supply of delicious salt-free casseroles in her freezer; another brought soup and smoothies and did her grocery shopping; others took her to doctors' appointments and helped with the medical paperwork. "I would never have asked them," she says. Luckily—and typically—they knew she needed help.

Not only do we have trouble asking for help, we even have trouble accepting it. Dr. Sara S. Auchincloss, a psychiatrist who specializes in people with serious afflictions and their families, has noticed that trait among her patients. It is a major "challenge for the woman to 'accept' what she needs from someone who is giving it to her, whether she asked or because they figured it out on their own." We have to learn to "tolerate it when people give care back to you," she says. Moreover, she has observed in her practice that we often set things up within our most intimate circle to ensure that the caregiving goes only one way. Many of Dr. Auchincloss's patients "have trained their nearest and dearest so successfully to expect to be taken care of, that when the woman herself gets sick, she's surrounded by a lot of dumbfounded people who have not got a *clue* what to do to begin to be able to take care of her."

Charlotte's experience with care getting prompted her, once she had recovered, to explore ways women in similar circumstances could get the support they needed but had so much trouble asking for. How could they establish the inter-dependence with others that they would need as crises occurred? She turned to The Transition Network (TTN), an organization she cofounded that has created a community for women over fifty who are exploring their next phase of life. She assembled a group to examine the problem by shar-ing their own experiences. One member admitted that she lay in bed for twenty-four hours with a broken leg so she wouldn't have to "impose on" her neighbors or her daughter, who was due to visit the day after her fall.

The group came up with a project they called the Caring Collaborative (CC). The premise is that women like Char-lotte and her TTN colleagues will never feel comfortable *ask-ing* for the occasional help they will need to "age in place." But they are very comfortable *offering* help to someone else. By joining a time bank, a participant earns care-getting credits—for when she needs it—by providing her services to another member. Members go through an orientation in which they are instructed on such issues as privacy and how to perform certain tasks (and how *not to* perform others, such as changing bandages or handling pills). A coordinator keeps track of members' locations, special strengths, and rel-evant experiences.

Caroline was one of the first to put the Caring Collabora-tive to the test when she was (literally) hit by a truck. From the emergency room she called a fellow CC member, who immediately sent out an all points bulletin; more than twenty members rallied to Caroline's care and recovery. They also became a collective patient advocate, a role that is essential in a medical crisis. With their backup, Caroline was able to demystify and then defy a surgical procedure a doctor recommended. The team's research concluded that the operation was controversial and possibly unnecessary. The Caring Collaborative is a tribute to the notion that you can do unto yourself as you have been doing unto others—by continuing to do unto others.

CARE-DRAINING RELATIONSHIPS

In the same way that building comfortable interdependent and supportive relationships with others fosters strength and promotes recovery, breaking free of a toxic and dependent relationship is also an act of self-preservation—care getting—that fosters well-being. After years of smoker's cough, Jean was finally scared into quitting when a fellow addict had a sudden heart attack. Detox was tough, but after that, "the next challenge became less scary," she writes. "Within months of quitting smoking, I finally ended my thirteen-year dysfunctional relationship. It wasn't neat or clean. It was ugly and hurtful and it dragged out; but it was clear to me that it was over and I had the strength to make it so. The man I lived with said to me, much after the break-up when it had become less painful to talk to each other, 'I knew when you quit smoking that my days were numbered.'" The commitment to her own wellness that prompted her to end her poisonous relationship with cigarettes was the handwriting on the wall for the equally toxic relationship with her boyfriend. Shedding an unhealthy or stale involvement—such as a friendship with someone who holds you back or puts you down or lets you down or drains your emotional energy—is an act of renewal and rebalancing.

Like Jean, the wake-up call of getting sick forced Gabby to reconsider what she was getting back from her relationships. What she found was a toxic relationship with herself. The antidote was to redirect the exorbitant amount of energy she expended on undertakings that depleted that energy into a new direction that would be life-affirming. Her life had been tumultuous from the start: She ran off to Paris as a teen, worked as an actress in London, and finally settled in the Midwest, where she runs a large arts organization. By her midfifties Gabby was an Energizer Bunny out of control. Then she was diagnosed with diabetes. "The doctor read me the riot act," she recalls. "He said, 'You know, if you carry on like this, the amount of work you do and the high-stressed life you live—and if you keep putting on this weight—you're going to be dead in ten years.' That pulled me up short, because I really hadn't thought about it very much. I was working eighty hours a week, and had been year in and year out for ages and ages. And I thought, He's right, I have to stop."

Cutting back on her work was the obvious place to begin. She asked for and got a reduced schedule and an assistant. The freed-up hours were devoted to getting her body back. "I got myself a trainer and I started going to the gym, and losing weight." With this physical reformation in process, she couldn't avoid looking into her inner life. "I started internalizing my life more and really trying to figure out what I wanted to do." That was where the real care getting began.

To find a less stressful and frustrating way of life within the whirlwind she knew she thrived on, Gabby would have to identify and nurture the true passions that drove her phenomenal lust for life. Creativity was one. She went back to acting, and began to write poetry. Love was another. She made peace with her secure but sexless marriage and entered into a totally insecure but high-drama and passionate liaison with a "bad boy" fifteen years younger. "I don't know; I just don't know," she keeps saying as she describes what might be considered a reckless series of choices. To Gabby, though, all the changes have been exhilarating; the upheaval has "made my life very interesting. And it has certainly focused me on my interior life a lot." It wasn't the stress that had been killing her; it was being estranged from the wildness at her core.

Once we begin to "focus on the interior life," we get a glimpse of the truth that ultimately care getting is a solitary business. Elizabeth Cady Stanton, the brilliant and wise suffragist, wrote a famous essay describing what she called "The Solitude of Self." In it she argues for equal rights for women on the grounds that every human being is ultimately alone, and therefore every citizen—woman and man—needs access to any and all the resources society provides. At the time she wrote it, she was also looking back over her own long life, and that gives special poignancy to her words. "Each soul must depend wholly on itself," she writes. It would be nice, she concedes, if it were otherwise, if the self-sacrifice expected from women were universal, but there are limits to caretaking. "We may have many friends, love, kindness, sympathy and charity, to smooth our pathway in everyday life," Stanton concludes, "but in the tragedies and triumphs of human experience, each mortal stands alone." Confronting that primal human condition is where caregiving and care getting become one.

DOING UNTO OTHERS—REDUX

Once we encounter that Solitary Self, we find ourselves drawn to other solitary souls. "What I have discovered through all my searching, traveling, studying, questing, struggling, pain, and suffering," Heather wrote me, "is that everyone's journey is in some way similar to mine. It seems that we are all on the same voyage, just sailing different ships. Ships sailing on one ocean, the ocean of life."

A yearning to connect with the "ocean of life" becomes

more intense as we near the far shore. Erik Erikson, whose pioneering work identified the several stages of the life cycle, calls this stage "generativity." A common first sign is the vague but energizing desire to get rid of "things" and concentrate on what matters. What turns out to matter is different for each of us, but the driving impulse is for, in Erikson's words, "community and affiliation." Generativity, wrote George Vaillant, a student of Erikson's work, reflects a "capacity to be in relationships where one 'cares.'" In all senses of the word. Doing good—caregiving to humankind—expands the possibilities for engaging in what matters—what we care about—and feeling good about ourselves—care getting. This circle of generosity opens up a range of avenues to the New Intimacy.

You don't have to retreat to a Zen monastery in order to connect with humankind. The "unconditional love" that grandparents lavish on their grandchildren is a powerful expression of generativity. "I had no idea it would feel like this, that I would love them so much," wrote a friend when she forwarded a piece of cyberwisdom: "Your kids are becoming you . . . and you don't like them . . . but your grandchildren are perfect." Often mistaken for "doting," which suggests mindless adoration, a grandparent's love can become an affirmation of unwavering belief in the child's authentic self—a lifelong counterweight to the self-doubt and regret we all experience. Unlike a parent, who is often distracted, harassed, and impatient, a grandparent has the distance, the devotion, and the trustworthiness to establish a core of confidence and acceptance in a child that no one else can. Elisabeth Kübler-Ross, who became an authority on death and dying, was initially surprised to find that many of the people she tended to at the end of their lives would call out for a grandparent. She came to believe that they were remembering the first, and perhaps only, source of unconditional love they had known.

I don't have grandchildren yet, so I can only murmur "Oooh, how adorable!" when presented with a photograph of a splotchy baby or an ice-cream-smeared toddler or a gawky teenager in front of Notre Dame. But I am blown away by the vulnerability and delight I see in my friends. And the passion. As one told me, "When I know one of my grandchildren is about to call, I feel my heart beating wildly as if I am expecting a lover."

Allan Shedlin, who counsels men on fatherhood, is divorced and has three daughters and five grandchildren. When I asked him to describe the love he feels for them, he began by telling me about the time one of his daughters, who was expecting her second child, confessed that she was worried that she couldn't possibly love another child the way she did her first. He reassured her that parental love was not finite and expanded with each child. "Grandparenting," he went on, "is the same."

But there are some differences, he adds, particularly in the ways that the love for a grandchild resonates across generations. The first time he became a grandfather, he says, "I instantly became a generation older (as did my 'child'), and I immediately had something in common with that adult child that we never had before—we are both parents!" But, most miraculous of all, the love pool has deepened all the way around. "One of the greatest gifts of becoming a grand-parent is realizing that your adult children will at last have an inkling of the depth of parental love you have felt for them over the years." What makes the relationship even more intense, my friend Susan has found, is that "not only are you giving unconditional love—you are *getting* it!"

Establishing a healthy equilibrium of giving and getting in a relationship is an especially daunting undertaking when loving care itself is the issue. Even when one person is depen-dent on another, the give-and-take of loving interdependence is still possible, provided the caregiver can sustain a similar balance within herself. The Solitary Self is holding the scales. When a woman becomes a Giving Tree, she will topple sooner or later if she doesn't pay attention to the roots that keep her upright. In nature, the roots of a healthy tree extend about three times the branch spread; we owe ourselves the same kind of support. Care getting is about preserving, protecting, and defending that core where you go home to yourself, no matter what. Defending that core is doubly life-enhancing, because our most generous impulses are generated there too.

Chapter 10

How We Love Now

Once the realization is accepted that even between the
closest human beings infinite distances exist, a marvelous
living side by side can grow up for them, if they succeed
in loving the expanse between them, which gives them
the possibility of always seeing each other as a whole and
before an immense sky.

—Rainer Maria Rilke, *Letters to a Young Poet*

My friend Brenda prides herself on being a wet blanket (she
would say "realist"); she lives in a half-empty glass. So when I
told her what I was writing about—love at midlife—I was prepared for her response. "Yeah, right," she said sardonically.
"Lots of luck finding any." I have thought of her often as I
have been interviewing and writing. Brenda was widowed

twenty years ago but pursued her very successful and exciting career for a long time after that. Nowadays she shares her professional skills by teaching two courses and has discovered a passion (and talent) for painting. She has a devoted son, two grandchildren she sees often, and a large circle of intimate friends, several of whom are regular theater (another passion) companions. Her more casual social community is regularly refreshed when she travels on tours organized around her many interests; she is passionate and opinionated about books and politics. A few years ago, she had a frightening showdown with mortality when she was diagnosed with cancer, but she made it through with the unremitting support of those who love her. She now feels strong and is back to hiking and swimming. But if you comment on how full of meaning and love her life is, she will always give the same answer: "Yeah, but why can't you find a man for me?"

During many of the conversations about the range and depth of experiences that are expanding the notion of love and defining a New Intimacy for women like her, I thought of how her conception of love—mired in the narrow terms of an earlier life—made it impossible for her to enjoy how more than half full her glass was. As I write this last chapter, I find myself thinking, Brenda, this book's for you.

So, what have I learned about how we love now? That my hunches were right: The way we experience intimacy is different from earlier times in our lives. That we are nurturing it in relationships that might not have developed in the past. That we are finding the kind of fulfillment, trust, and delight in a widening universe of intimate connections that deserve to be called love. And, most of all, that we are discovering new dimensions of give-and-take in those relationships, because we are uncovering new resources for giving and taking within ourselves.

I was delighted to find lots of evidence of a New Intimacy, but I wasn't prepared for the diversity and energy and satisfaction that it is generating. I heard dramatic stories about reinvented relationships, the Real Thing (at last), and the empowering nature of experimentation, risk, and true-to-yourself demands. I was less surprised—given what I know about women in Second Adulthood—but still impressed by the self-contained independence and personal authority I encountered. I was also struck by how well each relationship fit into a particular woman's life, regardless of its depth or shallowness. Some women found just the level of intimacy they wanted, but many others were content with the overall balance of loving relationships in their lives despite—or because of—the fact that many of them were less than the Real Thing.

And I was absolutely stunned by the role the Internet has assumed in our Second Adulthood. In cyberspace we meet, we find, we experiment, we play, we pretend, we reach out, we care for, we share, we tell the truth, we try on personalities, we maintain intimacy, we establish intimacy. After hearing story after story of an Internet-enhanced relationship, I do believe that all the "postmenopausal zest" we are generating would be severely constricted were it not for the technology that we have embraced with such enthusiasm.

Because the New Intimacy is based on personal authenticity and expanded experience, examples of it span the spectrum—from the profoundly trusting bond with friends to the profound commitment to "giving back"; from the unconditional love for a grandchild to the devotion between partners that is necessarily conditional in order to leave breathing room for each of them; to the very conditional vulnerability of what Erica Jong famously dubbed "a zipless fuck." The crucial consideration is making an assessment of the interdependence that each relationship can sustain. And then going for it.

Like loving itself, "going for it" is a continual undertaking. Circumstances change. Our needs and courage and strength are not always at the same level. Nor is our health. And very little comes to those who stand and wait. Whether it is loving a long-term partner or wanting to get to know a new tennis partner better, the equation of holding our own and reaching out poses daily challenges. We used to think that once you fell in love you were home free. In our first adulthood we learned that was *so* not so. But in our Second Adulthood we are learning that freedom is not the end product of finding love but its ongoing and ever-changing gift.

I have found that "interdependent" is the clearest description of the measured and balanced relationship that characterizes the New Intimacy. It reflects give-and-take, respect and tolerance, trust and freedom, between the people involved. If the balance is off, the mutuality is lost, and they fall back into dependence and disappointment. The magic of such relationships comes from the truth between two people and their shared wonder at how they fit.

That interdependence applies across the board. Even, and especially, to sex. When I talked to women about that part of their lives, I found myself posing a question that appeared on an early *Ms.* magazine cover: "How's Your Sex Life? ☐ Better ☐ Worse ☐ I Forget." The big surprise was how many women chose "Better." They are doing it when they can with more abandon, more satisfaction, and less guilt than ever before. For many this was a bonus they had least expected from these years, given their dismay over their bodies and the popular assumption that erotic joy wanes with menopause. The same confidence, daring, and ability to speak up for oneself that makes Second Adulthood so exhilarating is definitely behind the sexual awakening and hot sex many women are experiencing.

MORE WARMTH THAN HEAT

Relationships that, aside from the sex, might have been considered tepid by our former standards are, to many, warm and comforting now. People who didn't catch our attention then are turning out to be our most trusted intimates now. Cynics might call that "settling for half a loaf." But acceptance, we are discovering, is the whole loaf. We accept the ups and downs of our days. We accept the flaws and limitations of others, and therefore don't trust them beyond what they are capable of. Most of all, we are accepting of ourselves. There isn't much to work with, we find, in what we lack or what we have missed. It is the moment that has the most to offer the way we love now.

As is so often the case, there is a lovely piece of brain research that backs up this shift from seeing the glass half empty to appreciating that it is half full. Recent studies have shown that in our age group the amygdala—the most primitive response center in the brain—makes an analogous chemical adjustment. Whereas when we are young, brain scans light up equally in response to likes and dislikes, as we age, the brain increasingly responds to likes while the dislikes hardly register at all; they are filtered out. The message is clear: Why waste time on what doesn't work when there is so much that does? Gone are the fantasies of being swept off our feet; the women who have fallen in love are flying high, but their feet remain on the ground. Gone are the debilitating efforts to force a relationship into a model that doesn't fit; the only model is the one that feels right. The New Intimacy is whatever feels warm and healthy and uplifting—to body, mind, or spirit.

THE NEW INTIMACY AND (REINVENTED) YOU

The New Intimacy is based on **who you are now**. You are no longer the self-doubting young woman who would have rejected the "right guy" had she met him earlier. You are no longer the working woman forced to make hard choices. You are no more the harassed parent who didn't have time to stop and think. Your circumstances have changed; your choices have changed; you have changed. Back in your twenties and thirties you wouldn't have been able to call upon the qualities that now enrich your midlife relationships. As one recently divorced woman of forty-five explained when I told her what I was writing about, it took the rupture of her marriage to begin to see herself as a person, "rather than part of a couple." She feels her expectations have become more realistic. "Knowing myself better has enabled me to make better choices, to know what I want or need and to ask for it, but also to know when either of us is asking too much."

It is about **risk taking**. With accumulated confidence from your first adulthood, you are now able to let go of the notion of controlling things and take the chance of failure or the unexpected. You can venture beyond your comfort zone. You can explore the possibilities offered by a technology that is transforming the way we share our secrets, make ourselves vulnerable, and express our desires.

It is about **finding, not losing, yourself** in a relationship. That may explain why for most of the women I talked to, having the confidence to set their own terms made for more, not less, sharing. Why long-standing couples are staying married because they are finding new resources for staying engaged. And why some women are even reveling in the absence of formal attachments. Even when caregiving becomes a priority, it can still be of the doing-unto-yourself variety if you keep yourself in the picture.

It is about **second chances**. A review of your relationships—including family, friends, children, as well as lovers—is an opportunity for achieving more authenticity and clarity—and shedding resentment and disappointment. As a single forty-eight-year-old woman who likes things just the way they are put it, "I am in a relationship that doesn't 'need' but 'wants'—a relationship of mutual respect," adding with disbelief and wonder, "Who'd 'a thunk it."

And it is about **letting go**—of inhibitions, leftover "baggage" from past relationships, unrealistic expectations. And about reevaluating old priorities—children, habits, relatives, hobbies—and incorporating what still matters into the life you are building. Even in the most intimate relationships, there is much to let go of. "There may be things you want to share and it's just not a possibility," says Beth, a divorced fifty-year-old lawyer who feels that her current expectations are more in keeping with the limitations on sharing between two self-defined individuals. "He has his priorities, I have mine; so you have to figure out how to balance them."

It is—yes, Brenda—about **the glass half full**. The New Intimacy begins with acceptance—of who you are, how you look, and your worthiness to be loved. And the limitations of time. "Both sadness and happiness, but sadness more, are related to the fact that nothing of all this will endure for long," writes Carolyn Heilbrun. She goes on to describe an experience "unique to one's later years, of a swift, mysterious wave of happiness. . . . I cannot remember a time before my sixties, when the consciousness of happiness would sweep over me and, like a shower of cold water when one is desperately overheated, offer me a passing sensation very close to glee." Glee!

Finally it is about **finding a "peaceful place"** where the conflicts between past and present, love and work, who you are and who you thought you should be, are reconciled. Long-term marriages become less fraught and "bad boys" lose their appeal. Solitude becomes more comfortable. It is where the self-awareness and sense of mastery that we have achieved are directed at shaping a good life. And it is where the New Intimacy is celebrated.

The bottom line is that we are not too old to love in countless fulfilling and joyous ways, precisely because we are just old enough to know what love is—and what it is not. We have shed the notion that love is a gift from the gods, but accept with gratitude and a freewheeling delight the gifts each relationship brings.

Acknowledgments

Thanks to my husband, Bob, for his heroic crusade against *mush* in my writing and thinking. And to Wendy Wolf, whose smart comments pinpointed the many other lapses. Also Karin Lippert, another astute reader, who understands how important the Internet is to our generation and has assembled the Resources list of Web sites for this book. Steve Rubin's offer of an ideal work space made procrastination (almost) impossible. And, always and forever, I count on my "circle of trust" to guide and support my efforts.

Bibliography

Alboher, Marci. *The Encore Career Handbook: How to Make a Living and Make a Difference in the Second Half of Life.* New York: Workman Publishing, 2013.

Angier, Natalie. *Woman: An Intimate Geography.* New York: Anchor Books, 2000.

Applewhite, Ashton. *Cutting Loose: Why Women Who End Their Marriages Do So Well.* New York: HarperPerennial, 1998.

Apter, Terri. *Secret Paths: Women in the New Midlife.* New York: W. W. Norton & Company, 1995.

Bateson, Mary Catherine. *Composing a Further Life: The Age of Active Wisdom.* New York: Knopf, 2010.

Blum, Deborah. *Sex on the Brain: The Biological Differences Between Men + Women.* New York: Penguin Books, 1997.

Brizendine, Louann, M.D. *The Female Brain.* New York: Morgan Road Books, 2006.

Butler, Robert N., M.D., and Myrna I. Lewis, Ph.D. *The New Love and Sex After 60.* New York: Ballantine Books, 2002.

Carstensen, Laura L., Ph.D. *A Long Bright Future: An Action Plan for a Lifetime of Happiness, Health, and Financial Security.* New York: Broadway Books, 2009.

Bibliography

Civin, Michael. *Male Female e-mail: The Struggle for Relatedness in a Paranoid Society*. New York: Other Press, 2000.

Clinton, Hillary Rodham. *Living History*. New York: Simon & Schuster, 2003.

Coontz, Stephanie. *Marriage, a History*. New York: Penguin Books, 2006.

Dubois, Ellen Carol, ed. *The Elizabeth Cady Stanton–Susan B. Anthony Reader*. Foreword by Gerda Lerner. Boston: Northeastern University Press, 1992.

Ferris, Amy. *Marrying George Clooney: Confessions from a Midlife Crisis*. Berkeley, CA: Seal Press, 2009.

Fishel, Diedre, and Diana Holtzberg. *Still Doing It: The Intimate Lives of Women Over 60*. New York: Avery, 2008.

Fisher, Helen. *The First Sex: The Natural Talents of Women and How They Are Changing the World*. New York: Ballantine Books, 1999.

——. *Anatomy of Love: A Natural History of Mating, Marriage, and Why We Stray*. New York: Random House, 1992.

Fisher, Renee, Joyce Kramer, and Jean Peelen. *Invisible No More: The Secret Lives of Women Over 50*. New York: iUniverse, 2005.

Fisher, Joan. *Better Than I Ever Expected: Straight Talk About Sex After Sixty*. Emeryville, CA: Seal Press, 2006.

Fonda, Jane. *Prime Time: Love, Health, Sex, Fitness, Friendship, Spirit: Making the Most of your Life*. New York: Random House, 2011.

Freedman, Marc. *The Big Shift: Navigating the New Stage Beyond Midlife*. New York: Public Affairs, 2011.

Gilligan, Carol. *The Birth of Pleasure*. New York: Knopf, 2002.

——. *Kyra: A Novel*. New York: Random House, 2008.

Goldman, Connie. *Late Life Love: Romance & New Relationships in Later Years*. Minneapolis, MN: Fairview Press, 2006.

Hanauer, Cathi, ed. *The Bitch in the House: 26 Women Tell the Truth about Sex, Solitude, Work, Motherhood, and Marriage*. New York: William Morrow, 2002.

Hanover, Donna. *My Boyfriend's Back: Fifty True Stories of Reconnecting with a Long-Lost Love.* New York: Plume, 2005.

Heilbrun, Carolyn G. *The Last Gift of Time: Life Beyond Sixty.* New York: Ballantine Books, 1997.

Heyn, Dalma. *The Erotic Silence of the American Wife.* New York: Turtle Bay Books, 1992.

Katie, Byron. *I Need Your Love—Is That True? How to Stop Seeking Love, Approval, and Appreciation and Start Finding Them Instead.* New York: Three Rivers Press, 2005.

Fels, Anna. *Necessary Dreams: Ambition in Women's Changing Lives.* New York: Pantheon Books, 2004.

Kenison, Katrina. *The Gift of an Ordinary Day: A Mother's Memoir.* New York: Grand Central, 2010.

Lawrence-Lightfoot, Sara. *The Third Chapter: Passion, Risk, and Adventure in the 25 Years After 50.* New York: Farrar, Straus and Giroux, 2009.

Legato, Marianne J., M.D. *Eve's Rib: The New Science of Gender-Specific Medicine and How It Can Save Your Life.* New York: Harmony Books, 2002.

Lewis, Thomas, M.D., Fari Amini, M.D., and Richard Lannon, M.D. *A General Theory of Love.* New York: Vintage Books, 2000.

Northrup, Christiane, M.D. *The Wisdom of Menopause: Creating Physical and Emotional Health and Healing During the Change.* New York: Bantam Books, 2001.

Offill, Jenny, and Elissa Schappell, eds. *The Friend Who Got Away: Twenty Women's True-Life Tales of Friendships That Blew Up, Burned Out, or Faded Away.* New York: Doubleday, 2005.

Ogden, Gina, Ph.D. *The Heart & Soul of Sex: Making the Isis Connection.* Boston: Trumpeter, 2006.

Paley, Grace. *Begin Again: Collected Poems.* New York: Farrar, Straus and Giroux, 2001.

——. *Fidelity: Poems.* New York: Farrar, Straus and Giroux, 2008.

Price, Joan. *Naked at Our Age: Talking Out Loud About Senior Sex.* Berkeley, California: Seal Press, 2011.

Reily, Stephen, and Carol Osborn. *Vibrant Nation: What Boomer Women 50+ Know, Think, Do & Buy.* LaVergne, TN: VibrantNation.com., 2010.

Rentch, Gail, with The Transition Network. *Smart Women Don't Retire—They Break Free: From Working Full-time to Living Full-time.* New York: Springboard Press, 2008.

Sanford, Jenny. *Staying True.* New York: Ballantine Books, 2010.

Schwalbe, Robert, Ph.D. *Sixty, Sexy, and Successful: A Guide for Aging Male Baby Boomers.* Westport, CT: Praeger, 2008.

Sedlar, Jeri, and Rick Miners. *Don't Retire, Rewire! 5 Steps to Fulfilling Work That Fuels Your Passion, Suits Your Personality, and Fills Your Pocket.* New York: Alpha Books, 2003.

Sheehy, Gail. *Passages in Caregiving: Turning Chaos into Confidence.* New York: William Morrow, 2010.

——. *Sex and the Seasoned Woman: Pursuing the Passionate Life.* New York: Ballantine Books, 2007.

Trafford, Abigail. *As Time Goes By: Boomerang Marriages, Serial Spouses, Throwback Couples, and Other Romantic Adventures in an Age of Longevity.* New York: Basic Books, 2009.

Upham, Emily W., and Linda Gravenson, eds. *In The Fullness of Time: 32 Women on Life After 50.* New York: Atria, 2010.

Vaillant, George, M.D. *Aging Well: Surprising Guideposts to a Happier Life from the Landmark Harvard Study of Adult Development.* Boston: Little, Brown and Company, 2002.

Viorst, Judith. *Necessary Losses: The Loves, Illusions, Dependencies, and Impossible Expectations That All of Us Have to Give Up in Order to Grow.* New York: The Free Press, 2002.

Walbert, Kate. *A Short History of Women.* New York: Scribner, 2009.

Whyte, David. *The Three Marriages: Reimagining Work, Self and Relationship.* New York: Riverhead Books, 2009.

RESOURCES

AARP

www.aarp.org

Founded by Ethel Percy Andrus fifty years ago, the largest nonprofit membership organization in the United States working to enhance the quality of life for people fifty and over. The Web site is a comprehensive resource for information on health, wellness, sexuality, economic security, work, personal growth, relationships, entertainment, travel, and technology. Links to *AARP The Magazine, AARP VIVA,* TV and radio programs, blogs, and bulletins add to the site's information-rich experience.

ADMINISTRATION ON AGING

www.aoa.gov

An agency created to serve a growing senior population, providing access to a national network of home- and community-based services.

AGING ABUNDANTLY

www.agingabundantly.com

A Web site offering "Midlife Empowerment for Women." A place for women to gather to share thoughts, concerns, hopes, and dreams and to support one another in making the most of the second half of life. The site features experts on Health and Wellness, Family Life and Relationships, Hobbies and Interests, and Inspiration and Making a Difference.

AMAZINGWOMENROCK.COM

A popular destination for women created by Susan Macaulay, who believes every woman is special in her own way and has a story to tell and that we are all connected. The global community celebrates women of every age because they believe women tend not to blow their own horns. The online posts, videos, and tips cover everything from dance to food, music, science, and sex.

ASA/AMERICAN SOCIETY ON AGING

www.asaging.org

A multidisciplinary membership organization of researchers, practitioners, educators, and businesspeople providing resources on aging-related issues through the Aging in America Conference, Web seminars, continuing education programs, and a groundbreaking LGBT Aging Resources Clearinghouse.

BA50: BETTER AFTER 50

www.betterafter50.com

"Real Women—Real Stories, A Weekly Online Magazine." Women talking to one another about shared experiences—not talking *at* one another. "We're old enough—and wise enough—to approach the challenges and promise of mid-life with positive energy."

BLUE THONG SOCIETY

www.bluethongsociety.com

BTS chapters meet regularly in cities across the United States to plan outrageous outings, festive get-togethers, and fabulous efforts on behalf of the charitable causes they support. A sassy group of women with youthful spirits who want to connect both socially and philanthropically.

CARE.COM

www.care.com

A site for families and care providers to connect, share experiences, get advice, and find local resources. It features articles, expert advice, blogs, and specific caregiving guides for adults and seniors, and has a search capability by state and town.

CAREGIVER CREDIT CAMPAIGN

www.caregivercredit.org

Recognizing the importance and value of unpaid and underpaid care work inside and outside the home, this organization seeks to convert the Child Tax Credit to a Caregiver Tax Credit, covering care of adults and children, making it fully refundable and "Mommy Neutral," and increasing the value of the credit so it resembles the actual cost of giving care.

CARP, A NEW VISION OF AGING FOR CANADA
www.carp.ca

A national nonprofit membership and advocacy organization that is focused on financial security, pension and health-care reform, support for family caregivers, response to elder abuse, and freedom from ageism and discrimination of all kinds for people forty-five and over. It's a member of the Zoomer media family of Web sites: Zoomermag.com, 50plus.com, Zoomersingles.com, and others.

CENTERS FOR DISEASE CONTROL AND PREVENTION/HEALTHY AGING
www.cdc.gov/aging

Provides health information and resources on caregiving, clinical preventive services, the "Healthy Brain Initiative," cognitive impairment, mental health and aging, and Alzheimer's disease.

CIVIC VENTURES
www.civicventures.org

A think tank for boomers, work and social purpose that introduced Encore.org to help people explore encore careers that serve the greater good. Programs include The Purpose Prize, a financial investment in exceptional people over sixty who are using their experience to transform our nation, Encore Fellowships, and awards to innovative community colleges that prepare people fifty and over for careers in education and health care.

THE DANA FOUNDATION
www.dana.org

Offers brain research news, general resources and a directory for seniors, Webcasts, periodicals, and information on Brain Awareness Week.

EILEEN FISHER, INC.
www.eileenfisher.com

The Eileen Fisher Leadership Grant Program for Women & Girls and the Business Grant Program for Women Entrepreneurs are designed to support women and girls through social initiatives, promote activism, and empower women around the globe.

ENCORE.ORG
www.encore.org

Encore careers combine purpose, passion, and a paycheck in the second half of life. The organization was founded by Marc Freedman, author of *The Big Shift* and CEO and founder of Civic Ventures. Encore provides information on educational programs to retrain adults, job listings, news about expanding job fields, an online community, a directory of local organizations, social networking, and personal stories.

FABOVERFIFTY.COM
www.faboverfifty.com

Where the greatest generation of women (women over 50) network, blog, and share their favorite things—books, restaurants charities, beauty, style, and shops.

THE FAMILIES AND WORK INSTITUTE
www.familiesandwork.org

Founded in 1989, this is a nonprofit center for research on today's changing workforce, workplace, families, and communities.

FEISTY SIDE OF FIFTY
www.feistysideoffifty.com

A Web site celebrating "Baby Boomer Women 50 and Better" founded by Mary Eileen Williams, M.A., N.C.C., and author, who has more than twenty years' experience as a career/life counselor. She hosts a radio program that features well-known authors and experts on women in midlife with her special brand of feisty wisdom and humor.

FIRSTGOV FOR SENIORS
www.usa.gov/Topics/Seniors.shtml

A government-run Web site for seniors with links to a range of sites devoted to health, education, training, retirement planning, tax assistance, work, volunteer opportunities, travel, and leisure.

FOUNDATION FOR WOMEN'S WELLNESS
www.thefww.org

FWW targets the void in women's medicine by funding ground-breaking research on prevalent diseases and health conditions where data on gender differences is scarce. Major areas of research include cardiovascular disease, leading female cancers, and the role of hormones during pregnancy and menopause. Research analysis is disseminated directly to women via its newsletter, Web site, and at gatherings of physician-researchers.

GRANDPARENTS.COM
www.grandparents.com

Dedicated to America's 70 million grandparents, this Web site fosters family connections, including suggestions of child-and-grandparent-friendly activities, lifestyle features, expert advice, and how-to information about blogging, photo sharing, and video-chat applications. It also features products and membership benefits for grandparents, boomers, and seniors.

GRANDPARENTS FOR SOCIAL ACTION
www.grandparentsforsocialaction.org

A nationwide movement of grandparents and active seniors learning and sharing their roots in social action with their grandchildren. It organizes events, social action workshops, and trips, and explores opportunities for fun and innovative ways that grandparents and grandchildren can bond and learn together to heal the world.

HUFF/POST50

www.huffingtonpost.com/fifty/

The best blogs and conversation on topics that matter most to baby boomers: health, retirement, love, sex, parenting, and grandparenting.

THE KINSEY INSTITUTE

www.kinseyinstitute.org

The Kinsey Institute works toward advancing sexual health and knowledge worldwide. It is a leader in scholarship, teaching, and interdisciplinary study of sexuality, gender, and reproduction. The institute has a wide range of resources and programs, including audio podcasts.

MEDLINEPLUS

www.nlm.nih.gov/medlineplus

Produced by the U.S. National Library of Medicine and National Institutes of Health, this site is updated daily with information on clinical trials, drugs, diseases, supplements, and wellness issues in language for the general population.

MORE MAGAZINE

www.more.com

A magazine and Web site celebrating women forty and older with features on beauty, careers, fashion, health, food, travel, reinvention, money, relationships, societal issues, menopause, dating, sex, and love.

MS. FOUNDATION FOR WOMEN
www.ms.foundation.org

A social justice foundation that builds women's collective power to ignite policy and culture change throughout the United States. The grant program enables organizations to advance women's grassroots solutions across race and class in four areas: building democracy, economic justice, ending violence, and women's health. The foundation is the creator of "Take Our Daughters and Sons to Work."

MS. MAGAZINE AND BLOG
www.msmagazine.com
www.msmagazine.com/blog

Award-winning magazine founded in 1972 and now published by the Feminist Majority Foundation, with articles on feminist news, culture, justice, media, arts, women's studies, health, politics, and work, extensive coverage of international women's issues, and a take-action center. The *Ms.* Feminist Wire and the *Ms.* blog provide ongoing international and national news coverage of women's issues.

NATIONAL ALLIANCE FOR CAREGIVING
www.caregiving.org

A national coalition of nonprofit organizations focused on family caregiving that works on strengthening state and local groups and improving the quality of life for families and care recipients.

NATIONAL COUNCIL FOR RESEARCH ON WOMEN
www.ncrw.org

A network of 120 action-based organizations and a leading research, policy, and advocacy center committed to improving the lives of women and girls. A video for NCRW's twenty-fifth anniversary highlights changes and their belief that research powers revolution—collaborative and transformative change. *The Real Deal* blog and Webinars bring a range of voices and issues together on the site.

NATIONAL WOMEN'S HEALTH NETWORK
www.nwhn.org

A national organization founded in 1975 to give women a greater voice within the health-care system. It is supported by individuals and organizations nationwide and works to ensure that women have self-determination in all aspects of their reproductive and sexual health, monitor how menopause is perceived and addressed, and establish universal access to health care that meets the diverse needs of women. The site features health alerts, blogs, and a newsletter; answers basic health questions; and provides resources and position papers.

NATIONAL WOMEN'S LAW CENTER
www.nwlc.org

An organization that champions law and policies that work for women and families, from equal pay to women's health, in Congress, courts, and communities. The center's "Reports & Toolkits" provide advocates with information on a wide range of issues, including home-based care, equal pay, women and poverty, and health care, and a blog has daily updates on issues of concern to women.

NEW OLD AGE BLOG/THE NEW YORK TIMES
www.newoldage.blogs.nytimes.com

An informative blog about new developments on aging, health, finances, and the relationships between parents and their adult children caring for them.

NEXT AVENUE
www.nextavenue.org

A PBS-affiliated website designed to reach America's 50+ population who want to keep growing, keep learning, and keep doing in the next phase of life. Covers everything from Money & Security to Work & Purpose to Caregiving.

NIA
www.nianow.com
www.nianewyork.com

A sensory-based movement practice that leads to health, wellness, and fitness. It empowers people of all shapes, sizes, and ages by connecting the body, mind, emotions, and spirit. The Nia Technique draws on the disciplines of martial arts, dance arts, and healing arts to reconnect you with the joy of being in your own body through moves that are easy and are accompanied by music that comes from all over the world.

NORTHRUP, CHRISTIANE, M.D.

www.drnorthrup.com

An international pioneer on women's health and wellness and a leading proponent of medicine and healing that acknowledges the unity of mind and body. She is also the author of the classic *Women's Bodies, Women's Wisdom* and *Menopause and Beyond: New Wisdom for Women*. This Web site features health news, radio interviews, blog, Q&A, health products, and a bookstore.

OMEGA

http://eomega.org

http://eomega.org/omega/womensinstitute/

The Omega Institute for Holistic Studies is a trusted source for wellness and personal growth. A nonprofit organization, it has pioneered in exploring, teaching, and embracing new ideas focused on integrating body, mind, spirit, and creativity. The Women's Institute at Omega created the acclaimed Women & Power: Our Time to Lead conference, dedicated to transforming power, fostering a paradigm shift from control over others to partnership with others.

OUR BODIES, OURSELVES

www.ourbodiesourselves.org

The Boston Women's Health Book Collective is the nonprofit public interest women's education, advocacy, and consulting organization started in 1970 with the first edition of *Our Bodies, Ourselves,* which inspired the women's health movement. *Our Bodies, Ourselves: Meno-*

pause includes comprehensive health information on menopause and midlife. The Women's Health Information & Resource Center on the site includes excerpts from their books, Web-exclusive content, links, resources, health news, and a section called "Growing Older."

PERSIMMON TREE

www.persimmontree.org

More than an online magazine and showcase for the creativity and talent of women over sixty, this is a treasure chest of fiction, nonfiction, poetry, and theater pieces, art, conversations, and delightful short takes. The work validates the editors' belief that many women are at the height of their creative abilities in their later decades. The rich array of literary, educational, author, and adviser Web sites—names familiar and ones to be discovered—make the site a literary library for women of all ages.

REAL WOMEN ON HEALTH

www.realwomenonhealth.com

A women's community created by women inspired to become their best health and wellness advocates. It is run by women in midlife who are facilitating a dialogue about well-being and having candid conversations about diet and exercise; sexual health; women's health resources; and, mind, spirit, and body connections. The focus is on helping women advocate for themselves as patients, consumers, caregivers, working women, and community leaders.

RED HAT SOCIETY

www.redhatsociety.com

A global society of women that supports and encourages women in their pursuit of fun, friendship, freedom, fulfilling a lifelong dream, and fitness. RHS is dedicated to reshaping the way women are viewed in today's culture. Women over fifty are known as "Red Hatters"; those under fifty, as "Pink Hatters." The site offers members a strong online communication tool to share stories, start local chapters, and access shopping discounts, services, and events.

"RETIREMENT"—OR WHAT NEXT?

www.retirementorwhatnext.com

Support programs for women over fifty who are making life changes, founded by Ruth Neubauer, MSW, and Karen Van Allen, MSW. Programs include support groups, consultations by phone, and workshops in a nurturing environment with expert facilitators and presentations.

SCHWARTZ, PEPPER, PH.D.

www.drpepperschwartz.com

A leading relationship expert, Dr. Schwartz developed the Personality Profiler exclusively for the committed adults seeking long-term relationships on PerfectMatch.com. A matching tool that can be used on or off the Internet, the Personality Profiler helps individuals identify their potential significant others. The author of fourteen books, including *The Great Sex Weekend, The Lifetime Love and Sex Quiz Book,* and *Everything You Know About Love and Sex Is Wrong,* she lectures nationally on relationship topics, women's issues, and communication between women and men.

SECONDACT.COM

The online magazine with a mission to inspire boomers to keep growing and going strong at every age. Includes daily posts on news, work, money, health and fitness, the good life, giving back, and their *Prime Time* blog.

SENIOR FRIEND FINDER
www.seniorfriendfinder.com

A seniors' dating service whose purpose is to make it as easy as possible to make connections for dating, friendship, and romance using the Internet. It also offers a free interactive magazine, where members contribute poems, essays, articles, and comments.

SENIORS FOR LIVING
www.seniorsforliving.com

A free service to help people research, evaluate, contact, and compare senior housing options for assisted, independent, and retirement living as well as Alzheimer's care, continuing care, and home care. The blog provides news, health information, tips, and tools for navigating senior life, health, and caregiving issues. A "Top 100 Senior Blogs & Web Sites" listing provides a wide array of resources: humor, technology, socializing, dating and sex, alternative lifestyles, money and retirement, senior veterans, employment, senior care, and housing.

SENIORMATCH.COM

www.seniormatch.com

A safe network for those fifty and over to meet as singles, activity partners, travel companions, or dream lovers. The site includes blogs, message boards, and forums where members share experiences, questions, date ideas, senior news, activism, health information, dating advice, and safety tips, and can chat with one another.

SENIORNET

www.seniornet.org

A membership nonprofit organization that is bringing computer technology and education into the lives of adults fifty and over through an online learning center throughout the United States that enables older adults to share their wisdom, connect with families, and create a dynamic community on the Web site.

SHE WRITES

www.shewrites.com

SheWrites is a community, virtual workplace, and emerging marketplace for women who write, with members from all fifty states who are leveraging social-media tools and harnessing women's collaborative power. More than 250 groups focus on writing, community and specific interest groups from boomers to bloggers, e-publishers, memoir writers, and procrastinators. The site provides access to Webinars, radio programs, forums, and author services for professionals and emerging authors, from coaching writers to career management.

SHRIVER, MARIA
www.mariashriver.com

A Web site informed by Maria Shriver's worldview, support of women, ideas, inspiration, and information dedicated to architects of change. Its goal is to promote activism and empower women through a range of activities and groundbreaking reports. The Minerva Awards honor remarkable women, the *Every Woman Is Divine* video inspires, and her groundbreaking reports, *Alzheimer's in America* and *The Shriver Report* are valuable resources.

SMITH COLLEGE, THE ADA COMSTOCK SCHOLARS PROGRAM
www.smith.edu
www.smith.edu/classdeans/adas_about.php

The program is named for Ada Louise Comstock, who graduated from Smith College in 1897, served as dean from 1912 to 1923, and from 1923 to 1943 was president of Radcliffe College. Ada Comstock Scholars are a remarkable and diverse group of women ranging in age from their twenties to their midsixties who come to Smith at a time when they sense an undefined and unfulfilled potential in themselves; they may be mature, but they are unsure.

SOCIETY FOR WOMEN'S HEALTH RESEARCH
www.womenshealthresearch.org

A national nonprofit organization doing research based on sex differences and dedicated to improving women's health through advocacy, education, and research. The Web site features information regarding health disorders that affect women predominantly or differently than men, and promotes the inclusion of women and minorities in clinical trials.

SOPHIA SMITH COLLECTION (SSC)
Women's History Archive at Smith College

An internationally recognized repository of manuscripts, archives, photographs, periodicals, and other primary sources in women's history. It was founded in 1942 to be the library's distinctive contribution to the college's mission. The collection's holdings document the historical experience of women in the U.S. and abroad from the colonial era to the present. Suzanne Braun Levine's papers from her years as editor of *Ms.* are there, along with those of other *Ms.* editors, including Gloria Steinem.

THIRDAGE.COM
www.thirdage.com

The leading online site focused on serving baby boomers. It provides information and insightful content on relationships and sex, family and friends, money and work, beauty and style, and travel and pastimes. "Aging Well" and the "Women's Health Center" include resources on common problems faced by boomers, there are community Q&A sections, and e-mail newsletters and alerts provide the latest news and articles about relationships and love.

THOMAS, MARLO
www.marlothomas.com

The latest project of Marlo Thomas, actor, producer, activist, author, and advocate for women, children, and families. The site is a conversation about women's real lives and features "live" interactive programs, called *Mondays with Marlo,* with experts and friends on topics from health, finance, and fashion to politics, humor, and technology.

THE TRANSITION NETWORK
www.thetransitionnetwork.org

A nonprofit national organization for women over fifty who join forces to successfully navigate life's transitions. Small group interactions, programs, and workshops inspire members to support one another and to continue a life of learning, engagement, and leadership in the world. Local chapters sponsor events, Peer Groups address special-interest areas, and the TTN Caring Collaborative is an innovative model for organizing care for an aging community.

VIBRANT NATION
www.vibrantnation.com

The leading online community for baby boomer women—a place where they connect and support one another on issues unique to life after fifty, including fashion, beauty, family, relationships, work, money, and sex. A resource and growing network of more than one hundred midlife bloggers, the site promotes off-line gatherings and publishes digital health and beauty content written by women experts.

VILLAGE TO VILLAGE NETWORK
www.vtvnetwork.org

A national network of grassroots organizations formed to serve and help seniors live independently in their communities and neighborhoods. Established to coordinate access to affordable services enabling seniors to lead safe, healthy, productive lives in their own homes by coordinating transportation, health and wellness programs, home repairs, social and education activities, and trips, villages are based on the needs of the community and do everything and anything that their members need. It's a model for a new community-based approach to aging.

WOMANSAGE
www.womansage.org

A nonprofit organization for boomer women who want an opportunity to reinvent themselves, find pathways to meet the challenges of aging, support groups of women, and learn fresh ways to assess their skills and talents. Founded by former syndicated columnist Jane Glenn Haas, the organization provides support through educational programs, networking, events, news, and social philanthropy.

WOMEN'S ENEWS.ORG

www.womensenews.org

A prize-winning nonprofit daily Internet-based news service cover-ing issues of concern to women and their allies, it is supported by its readers, events, foundations, and resale of its content. Freelance writers from around the world write on every topic—politics, reli-gion, economics, health, science, education, sports, and legislation—and are featured along with commentaries, monthly columns, and editorial cartoons by prominent journalists and advocates.

WOMEN'S HEALTH INITIATIVE

www.nhlbi.nih.gov/whi

An organization that reports on the ongoing findings of the Women's Health Initiative Hormone Therapy Trials, a fifteen-year research program to address the most common causes of death, disability, and poor quality of life in postmenopausal women—cardiovascular disease, cancer, and osteoporosis. It is one of the largest U.S. prevention studies of its kind established by the National Institutes of Health (NIH).

WOMEN'S MEDIA CENTER

www.womensmediacenter.com

A nonprofit progressive organization that makes women visible and powerful in the media to ensure that women's stories are told and voices are heard. Daily "Exclusive" news and issue features, "News Briefs," women experts on issues, a media training program, outreach online, and panels convened by the organization, along with grassroots campaigns, generate national attention and are bringing diversity into the media landscape.

ZOOMER MAGAZINE

www.zoomermag.com

Partnered with CARP, *Zoomer* magazine was created for "boomers with zip." This lifestyle publication relevant to Canadians forty-five and over is part of the Zoomer media family of Web sites, with entertaining and engaging content for women and men who embrace life with experience and confidence and aren't afraid of change.

Index

Index

Index

Index